Advancing Responsible Adolescent Development

Series Editor

Roger J. R. Levesque
Department of Criminal Justice
Indiana University
Bloomington, IN, USA

Brief Overview

This series advances disciplinary and multidisciplinary inquiry into the individual, social, biological, and institutional responses to adolescents and their development. It champions research that examines conditions that either stifle or enhance responsible development.

Description

Responsible adolescent development - one that is healthy, fulfilling, engaged, and respectful of one's self and others - requires responsive relationships with families, peers, neighbors, schools, community organizations, religious institutions, and other socializing systems. All these socializing influences reach optimal effectiveness when reinforced by appropriate social policies and norms at local, cultural, state, national, international and global levels. This series examines the wide variety of sources that shape responses to adolescents and responsible development. This series explores these complex sources by exhibiting theories, models, research studies, and symposia that examine multiple dimensions of adolescent development. Drawing from numerous disciplines, the series examines dimensions and experiences of adolescent development that contribute to responsibility (including irresponsibility) in multiple contexts and settings. The focus on multiple arenas of development necessarily encompasses the need to center on adolescents as well as on the conditions in which they live. Thus, the series publishes manuscripts that speak to issues adolescents face, but does not require that texts directly study adolescents themselves. Manuscripts may examine images and portrayals of adolescents through, for example, cultural assumptions of parenting, media depictions, religious groups' proselytizing, schooling's hidden curriculum, justice systems' presumptions, clinicians' interventions, and many other potential influences on adolescent development. The broadening of the disciplinary and multidisciplinary study of adolescence, however, does not mean that the series ignores core issues from adolescents' own perspectives, such as adolescents' experiences with significant others and with the wide variety of tasks, risks, and opportunities they encounter.

More information about this series at http://www.springer.com/series/7284

Rhonda Tabbah

Arab American Youth

Discrimination, Development, and Educational Practice and Policy

Springer

Rhonda Tabbah
Columbus, OH, USA

ISSN 2195-089X ISSN 2195-0903 (electronic)
Advancing Responsible Adolescent Development
ISBN 978-3-030-66803-7 ISBN 978-3-030-66804-4 (eBook)
https://doi.org/10.1007/978-3-030-66804-4

This Springer imprint is published by the registered company Springer Nature Switzerland AG
The registered company address is: Gewerbestrasse 11, 6330 Cham, Switzerland

"Dr. Tabbah has written a book that is well overdue... she provides a blueprint for moving forward in education as well as in policy development that can be transformative for Arab-American youth."

—Antoinette Miranda, Professor, School Psychology,
The Ohio State University

"This book is a valuable contribution given the nascent literature on the experiences of Arab youth and the significant impact of discrimination on their schooling."

—Desiree Vega, Associate Professor of School Psychology,
University of Arizona

I dedicate this book to my baby girl, Nadine, my inspiration for continuing to pursue my passion for research on Arab youth in America.

Preface

My passion for research on Arab youth in America began during my graduate school career in School Psychology at the Ohio State University. In courses that addressed multicultural issues, Arab cultures were minimally mentioned, if mentioned at all. As an Arab American myself, this pushed me to research why this was the case. As I delved into the literature, I was disappointed to find only a few literary pieces regarding Arab American youth. Moreover, the studies I did find were somewhat dated. Given the events of the terrorist attacks of 9/11 and the resulting backlash Arab American communities experienced, I felt that research on this group was imperative. Therefore, I made it my mission to pursue research with this ethnic group and attempt to increase the literature in the fields of education and psychology.

My mission began with my doctoral dissertation which examined development of Arab American youth in relation to their school experiences. My study sought to provide a voice for Arab youth. Their voices became a beacon for me to continue this research path and contribute to the knowledge on Arab youth in the American education system. I was able to publish several papers and present my evidence at conferences of the National Association of School Psychologists. Since then, an increase in research regarding Arab youth has emerged. This allowed me to contribute a narrative review of the literature, which led me to Professor Roger J.R. Levesque, the journal editor of *Adolescent Research Review*, who encouraged a proposal of this book on Arab youth in the education system. Without his support, this would not have been possible.

This book addresses the experiences of Arab youth in the American education system with the ultimate goal of serving as a tool for educators and providers to address the perils they face. The volume offers a thorough historical background of the Arab experience in America beginning with their immigration. Greater societal discrimination is discussed to provide context for school experiences. The importance of understanding this history lies in the fact that discrimination has been found to influence development. Therefore, the volume discusses the most relevant theories to Arab American youth followed by a narrative review of the research existing on this group. Research limitations are thoroughly presented alongside strategies to address these issues. The book concludes with a presentation regarding reform in education practice and policy with Arab American youth. It is my hope that this volume will aid in the improvement of school environment for Arab American youth to, consequently, foster healthy development.

My progress could not have been possible without several individuals who influenced me and supported my research career. I would like to acknowledge Drs. Antoinette Miranda, Joe Wheaton, and Kisha Radliff at the Ohio State University for fostering my research interests from the very beginning in graduate school. These amazing mentors helped me plant a seed that continues to flourish. Next, I would like to acknowledge Dr. Roger J.R. Levesque for his support and encouragement from the time of the proposal and throughout the development of this volume. His support, along with the support of the senior editor, Judy Jones, was integral in the conception of this manuscript. Finally, but definitely not least, support from my family was fundamental in the completion of this book. My parents, Isam and Sumayah, my niece, Zayna, and my sister, Ranya, thank you for helping with childcare. My husband, Hazem, thank you for believing in and encouraging me always. My niece, Maya, thank you for being my second eyes and taking the time to read my drafts. I am eternally grateful for you.

Columbus, OH, USA Rhonda Tabbah Ph.D.

About this Book

This book examines the implications of discrimination in Arab American youth with a focus on K-12 school systems. It begins with an introduction to Arab American youth and their experiences in the education system. The book follows with an overview regarding historical contributions of discrimination and the history of discrimination against Arabs in America, including the education system. It then presents relevant theoretical perspectives regarding discrimination and developmental processes. The book examines research specific to Arab American youth, identifies research limitations, and provides strategies on how to strengthen methodological approaches to better inform research, practice, and policy. It concludes by offering strategies for improving educational practice and policy and recommendations for interventions designed to enhance developmental health of Arab American youth in schools.

Key areas of coverage include:

- Arab American youth, development, and discrimination in America.
- Discrimination in the K-12 educational system.
- Self-concept, ethnic identity, well-being and discrimination among Arab American youth.

Arab American Youth is an essential resource for practitioners, researchers, educators, and related professionals as well as graduate students in school psychology, educational psychology, education, and related disciplines.

Contents

About the Author

Rhonda Tabbah, Ph.D. is a school psychologist currently engaging in independent research. She graduated with her doctorate in School Psychology from the Ohio State University in 2011. Dr. Tabbah practiced in the Columbus City School District intermittently for 5 years with her most recent assignment involving a combination middle-high school, which focused on multiculturalism and an international curriculum. As a bilingual, Arabic English–speaking school psychologist, Dr. Tabbah also worked with bilingual students and English language learners. Her work in a multicultural setting, along with her personal research, allowed Dr. Tabbah to exercise her passions, learn about diverse populations in her schools, and develop a skill set for culturally competent practices. Her research has focused on the experiences of Arab American adolescents in the school system, using this information for social justice reform and improving the quality and accuracy of multicultural curricula related to this subgroup. Dr. Tabbah is interested in development and strengthening of policies for social justice and building cross-cultural and intercultural relationships in the educational system.

An Introduction to Arab American Youth

Introduction

Arabs in America have historically faced discrimination, prejudice, and stereotyping, especially after 9/11. The impact of political injustice and ethnic hate crimes resulting from the attacks on Arab American families have shown to have dire consequences, especially for their youth in the education system. After the attacks, Arab American youth faced discrimination in the schools from their peers, teachers, and other staff members. Perpetual cultural misconceptions are evident throughout various facets of society and, therefore, have infiltrated the education system in America. Research demonstrates that all levels of the education system are impacted, including practice and policy. For example, stereotypes and misperceptions have manifested in discriminatory behaviors toward Arab youth from educators and peers. In addition, stereotypes and misconceptions of Arab cultures are evident in school curricula, which further perpetuates the problem. Therefore, reform of educational practice and policy relative to Arab American youth is imperative.

The purpose of this book is to examine the implications of discrimination on development—including ethnic identity and well-being—in Arab American youth. The importance of investigating ethnic identity in this population stems from evidence that high ethnic awareness may be protective against the development of a negative self-concept and may support a sense of psychological well-being in individuals who come from devalued ethnic groups (Mossakowski, 2003; Rivas-Drake, Hughes, & Way, 2008). The literature regarding this group is relatively scarce compared to other ethnic minority groups. Consequently, this volume discusses implications for future research directions in order to increase the body of evidence available and to strengthen methodological approaches to better inform research, practice, and policy. This book also offers recommendations for interventions designed to foster healthy development of Arab youth and strategies for improving educational practice and policy.

R. Tabbah, *Arab American Youth*, Advancing Responsible Adolescent Development, https://doi.org/10.1007/978-3-030-66804-4_1

To provide readers with context regarding the book's focus, this chapter introduces a preview of the various factors that are critical to consider in the experiences of Arab American youth, beginning with the historical contributors of discrimination. Because schools do not exist in a vacuum, stereotypes and discrimination across mainstream society must also be considered to truly understand their experiences. School systems may serve as either a risk factor or a protective factor in adolescent development, depending on the climate. In the case of Arab American youth, research demonstrates that school environment is, indeed, related to various developmental outcomes. Therefore, educators and school providers must strive to create a positive, inclusive environment for Arab American youth. This chapter concludes with a description of the content entailed in each chapter of this volume.

Arab American Youth, Development, and Discrimination in Education Systems

There is a large and ever-growing population of Arab Americans in the United States (Cainkar, 2016). Be that as it may, researchers have long considered this group as an invisible minority (e.g., Suleiman, 2000), at least up until the 9/11 terrorist attacks. Arab cultures in America have been historically misrepresented through media and various other sources (Awad & Amayreh, 2016). However, since the 9/11 terrorist attacks, negative images of Arabs and their cultures have permeated the media and American society as a whole (Harb, 2016). Arabs were further portrayed in the media as terrorists, the common enemy, and as "other" (Abu El-Haj, 2006). One of the most common misconceptions, for example, is the interchangeability of the terms "Arab" and "Muslim" (Al-Hazza & Lucking, 2005). Arab American is a category which encompasses individuals with diverse religious practices among various demographic factors, such as racial, national, dialectal, and political backgrounds (Hakim-Larson & Menna, 2016). In fact, the Arab American population is largely Christian (Amer & Kayyali, 2016). Therefore, this particular misconception erases the heterogeneity of this ethnic group (Suleiman, 2000).

More recent events involving the Arab Spring and the rise of ISIS in Iraq and Syria have brought to the forefront and further complicated socio-political issues in the media (Harb, 2016). As a consequence of the attacks in Paris, France in 2015 by ISIS, the American Arab Anti-Discrimination Committee (ADC) has been working diligently to dispel misconceptions being conveyed in the media (ADC, 2015). Furthermore, the Arab American Institute (AAI) conducted a recent poll revealing that views have only increased in negativity since their previous survey study in 2010, suggesting that there continue to be persistent and hostile portrayals of Arabs and Muslims in America (AAI, 2015).

The historical standard of misrepresentation of Arab cultures in America leads researchers to suggest that there is an expected risk to developmental processes in Arab American youth within multicultural society (Al-Hazza & Bucher, 2010).

There is evidence that negative perceptions and stereotypes in mainstream United States media have led to a hostile environment and various forms of discrimination for Arabs in America (Bayoumi, 2009). Incidents of hate against Arabs in America did occur prior to 9/11 albeit rather infrequently. However, following the attacks, the number of incidents surged (Ibish, 2001). The latest report from the American Arab Anti-Discrimination Committee (ADC, 2011) stated a recent string of deaths by suicide as a result of acts of discrimination and bullying in the K-12 system.

Negative perceptions have also been validated in empirical research. For example, Wray-Lake, Syvertsen, and Flanagan (2008) used open-ended questionnaires to collect data on sensitivity to images as enemies of America, experiences of prejudice and discrimination, and times when adolescent participants felt American. Results indicated that regardless of ethnic background, Arabs were nominated as enemies of America more than any other category. Over 69% of the Arab sample believed that Arabs in general or a specific Arab group were portrayed as enemies of America. Furthermore, out of the 93 Arab participants, 63 reported experiencing prejudice where almost half were related to "being physically or outwardly identified as Arab" (p. 89). Consequently, adolescents of Arab descent in America are expectedly forming their identities in an environment surrounded by racism and prejudice with a keen awareness of the publics' low regard for the Arab American community (Read, 2008). The experiences of Arab youth in America as a devalued ethnic group warrants investigation of encounters regarding developmental processes, including ethnic identity and well-being.

Experiences of discrimination have been linked to the development of self-concept (Moradi & Hasan, 2004), a relationship known as the stigma hypothesis. The stigma hypothesis states that the internalization of stigma or minority status leads to lower self-concept in minority groups (Twenge & Crocker, 2002). The status of being a minority becomes internalized with experiences of prejudice and discrimination. According to symbolic interaction theorists, these experiences would be considered negative social interactions with others. As a result, members of minority groups become affected psychologically (Kenny & McEachern, 2009). A possible protective factor in this process may be ethnic identity.

Experiences of discrimination have been linked to the formation of both individual and collective identity, especially for adolescents (Wray-Lake et al., 2008). Many youth become preoccupied with the judgments of others as they search for self-identity (Harter, 1999). Experiences of discrimination can often play a catalytic role in adolescents' examination of what it means to be a member of a marginalized ethnic group. Negative experiences with the majority may lead to feelings of rejection, which could result in increased identification with their own devalued ethnic group to preserve feelings of belonging and maintain self-esteem, a process defined as the rejection-identification model (Branscombe, Schmitt, & Harvey, 1999). The rejection-identification model is based on the research of Branscombe et al. (1999) who found a direct, positive relationship between self-perceived discrimination and increased ethnic identity among African Americans. The model recognizes that discrimination can negatively affect well-being, but this can be counteracted through increased ethnic identification.

For adolescents, it is particularly important to examine the school climate since this is where they spend a significant portion of their day. The school system delivers essential means of socialization and is critical to youth development (Ajrouch, Hakim-Larson, & Fakih, 2016). In addition to overall well-being, several studies have shown that ethnic identity is significantly related to and a significant predictor of academic achievement in ethnic minority youth (Harper & Tuckman, 2006; Worrell, 2007). An interplaying factor in this relationship may be perceptions of discrimination or stereotyping of ethnic minorities in the school setting.

Haboush and Alyan (2016) reported that school environments became less tolerant of Arab American youth following the 9/11 terrorist attacks. Ajrouch and Awad (2019) found that Arab American youth are not likely to seek help from adults in schools because they may be the source of bias or perpetuate negative stereotypes of Arab Americans. Stereotypes and misperceptions of Arab cultures and history are also evident in the school curriculum (Ajrouch & Awad, 2019). Wingfield and Karaman (2009) discussed the potential negative effects of these types of experiences:

> They may find that the message about the Arab world in school conflict with the values and traditions passed on at home. The images of Arabs which are conveyed in the classroom may have nothing in common with their relatives and experiences at home or their friends and relatives in the neighborhood, church/mosque, or elsewhere. They also find their peers to be influenced by negative and inaccurate images and preconceptions about the Arab heritage. Obviously these circumstances lead to hurtful experiences…. Like other ethnics, Arab Americans frequently encounter negative stereotypes disguised in the form of "humor." When they object, they are told that the derogatory comments were "not meant to be taken seriously." Today there should be greater public awareness and acknowledgement that not taking the identity of others seriously is just another form of racism.

Therefore, the purpose of this book is to examine the implications of discrimination on development in Arab American youth and to, ultimately, inform on educational policy and practice reform regarding this population. Schools tend to reproduce the structures that exist in the society in which they operate. Therefore, it is necessary to situate the experiences of Arab American adolescents in schools within the greater context of the history of Arab Americans in the United States and the trends of discrimination that have existed prior to and following the terrorist attacks of 9/11. In order to truly understand the Arab experience in America, it is critical to learn their history with immigration to the United States, as well as the various issues regarding culture, race, and identity this group has encountered throughout history beginning with their immigration in the 1800s. Chapter "Arab American Youth and Historical Contributors of Discrimination" leads this discussion. Given the inconsistencies of racial categorization of Arabs in America, researchers argue that this group, while currently identified by the United States government as white, has historically been "white, but not quite." This dilemma has caused confusion and inconsistencies with self-identification throughout and within Arab American communities and individuals when it comes to race and identity. Additionally, this group has experienced discrimination similar to other ethnic minority groups who are not characterized as "white." Being labeled as white by the government also excludes them from affirmative action. These issues have been found to relate to a range of reactions to discrimination experiences within the Arab communities. As discussed in chapter "Arab American Youth and Historical Contributors of Discrimination", researchers argue that discrimination experiences throughout history are related to cultural conditioning of the mainstream public through negative portrayals and perceptions of Arab people and their cultures in the corporate media. This opens up an exploration of the Arab American experience with discrimination in both pre- and post-9/11 eras in chapters "Arab American Youth and Discrimination in the Pre-9/11 Era" and "Arab American Youth and Discrimination Post-9/11", respectively.

Chapter "Arab American Youth and Discrimination in the Pre-9/11 Era" illustrates a long history of discrimination experienced in the Arab American community beginning with their immigration to the United States in the 1800s. Stereotypes throughout the media were also rampant through sources such as television and motion pictures. Chapter "Arab American Youth and Discrimination in the Pre-9/11 Era" describes how Arabs have historically been invisible in one moment and then extremely visible in the next, even prior to 9/11. The chapter exemplifies how the same negative portrayals, misconceptions, and discrimination were evident prior to 9/11, and how 9/11 was only a turning point where all of these issues were magnified. Chapter "Arab American Youth and Discrimination in the Pre-9/11 Era" also demonstrates how stereotypes and discrimination of Arabs are deeply rooted in American society.

Chapter "Arab American Youth and Discrimination Post-9/11" continues the journey of the various experiences Arabs in America have encountered post-9/11 including hate crimes, violence, civil liberties being infringed upon, racial profiling, and law enforcement misconduct. These experiences reportedly occurred in various public and private settings, including schools. The dialogue demonstrates how immigration and racial factors discussed in chapter "Arab American Youth and Historical Contributors of Discrimination" come into play with discrimination against this group. Chapters "Arab American Youth and Historical Contributors of Discrimination" through "Arab American Youth and Discrimination Post-9/11" provide the context necessary to fully understand the experiences of Arabs in American society, and open the door for a deeper examination of their experiences within the education system.

Chapter "Arab American Youth and Discrimination in the Education System" continues the discrimination dialogue with a focus on adolescent experiences in the education system. It presents how cultural misrepresentation and/or lack thereof in the multicultural paradigm have infiltrated educational environments. The dialogue includes the various misconceptions and cultural exclusion that have contributed to prejudice and discrimination in the school systems.

Chapter "Developmental Theories Relevant to Arab American Youth" builds on the presented overview of Arab American experiences to introduce various theories encompassing the relations between discrimination and adolescent development. Several theories exist in the literature regarding these relationships, including the ecological model of human development, symbolic interaction theory, stigma hypothesis, social identity theory, and rejection-identification model. The chapter begins with a discussion on Bronfenbrenner's ecological model of human development and how discrimination infiltrates systemic levels influencing development. Then, youth identity development is addressed with a focus on ethnic identity. Research, and/or the lack thereof, regarding ethnic identity development as a construct with Arab American youth is presented. Theories involving discrimination influences on identity include social identity theory and the rejection identification model. Next, the process of self-concept development is discussed along with the research available regarding this development in Arab American adolescents. Theories involving discrimination are presented, including symbolic interaction theory and stigma hypothesis. The chapter concludes with a presentation of the various developmental outcomes of discrimination found specifically in the school system, including psychological, behavioral, social, academic, and physical consequences.

Subsequently, chapter "Discrimination and Developmental Processes in Arab American Youth" presents a narrative review on research findings specific to Arab American adolescents regarding developmental outcomes when faced with discrimination. The review includes research conducted in various settings, including the school systems. The reason being that, as stated earlier, schools do not exist in a vacuum.

Chapter "Discrimination and Developmental Processes: Bridging the Research Gap on Arab American Youth" examines the existing research on the development and discrimination in Arab American youth for common methodological limitations and gaps found within and across studies. It provides strategies for strengthening methodology for future researchers to consider and for increasing empirical evidence to better inform educational practice and policy with Arab American adolescent populations.

Conclusively, Chapter "Transforming Education Practice and Policy for Arab American Youth" focuses on the implications of the existing research and reform of educational practice and policy relevant to Arab American youth. The chapter examines the existing research for common themes regarding areas of the school environment that need addressed. The dialogue then suggests strategies to implement for each of the areas identified. The text includes a detailed overview of important factors of Arab American cultures to help build cultural awareness for educators and school practitioners. These are considered general guidelines, as each family will have its own individual characteristics. Then, the process of developing cultural competence is presented with regard to Arab cultures. This is followed by a discussion regarding various interventions that can be implemented to address peer and teacher relationships. Recommendations are then provided for education reform to include and/or accurately represent Arabs and Arab Americans at all levels, including multicultural curricula. Chapter "Transforming Education Practice and Policy for Arab American Youth" concludes with a presentation on the process for implementing interventions with Arab American adolescents in school to address developmental outcomes with a focus on the aspects of mental health. In combination, this book serves as a reference to better understand the experiences of Arab American youth, how these experiences impact their development, and what educators and school providers can do to better serve them to foster healthy development.

References

AAI. (2015). *American attitudes toward Arabs and Muslims: 2015*. Retrieved September 15, 2019, from http://www.aaiusa.org/american_attitudes_toward_arabs_and_muslims_2015

Abu El-Haj, T. R. (2006). Race, politics, and Arab American youth: Shifting frameworks for conceptualizing educational equity. *Educational Policy, 20*, 13–34. https://doi.org/10.1177/0895904805285287.

ADC. (2011). *The 2010 ADC legal report: Legal advocacy and policy review*. Washington, DC: American Arab Anti-Discrimination Committee.

ADC. (2015). *Refuting the myths in the Syrian and Iraqi refugee debate: ADC separates fact from fiction*. Retrieved September 20, 2019, from http://www.adc.org/2015/11/refuting-the-myths-in-the-syrian-and-iraqi-refugee-debate-adc-separates-fact-from-fiction/

Ajrouch, K. J., & Awad, G. H. (2019). An ecological approach to childhood prejudice: The case of Arab Americans. In H. E. Fitzgerald, D. J. Johnson, D. B. Qin, F. A. Villarruel, & J. Norder (Eds.), *Handbook of children and prejudice: Integrating research, practice, and policy* (pp. 147–159). Cham, Switzerland: Springer.

Ajrouch, K. J., Hakim-Larson, J., & Fakih, R. (2016). Youth development: An ecological approach to identity. In M. M. Amer & G. H. Awad (Eds.), *Handbook of Arab American psychology* (pp. 91–102). New York: Routledge.

Al-Hazza, T., & Bucher, K. T. (2010). Bridging a cultural divide with literature about Arabs and Arab Americans. *Middle School Journal, 41*, 4–11. https://doi.org/10.2307/23047567.

Al-Hazza, T., & Lucking, B. (2005). The minority of suspicion: Arab Americans. *MultiCultural Review, 14*, 32–38.

Amer, M. M., & Kayyali, R. A. (2016). Religion and religiosity: Christian and Muslim faiths, diverse practices, and psychological correlates. In M. M. Amer & G. H. Awad (Eds.), *Handbook of Arab American psychology*. New York: Routledge.

Awad, G. H., & Amayreh, W. M. (2016). Discrimination: Heightened prejudice post 9/11 and psychological outcomes. In M. M. Amer & G. H. Awad (Eds.), *Handbook of Arab American psychology* (pp. 63–75). New York: Routledge.

Bayoumi, M. (2009). *How does it feel to be a problem?: Being young and Arab in America*. New York: Penguin.

Branscombe, N. R., Schmitt, M. T., & Harvey, R. D. (1999). Perceiving pervasive discrimination among African Americans: Implications for group identification and well-being. *Journal of Personality and Social Psychology, 77*(1), 135–149. https://doi.org/10.1037/0022-3514.77.1.135.

Cainkar, L. (2016). Race and racialization: Demographic trends and the process of reckoning social place. In M. M. Amer & G. H. Awad (Eds.), *Handbook of Arab American psychology* (pp. 19–33). New York: Routledge.

Haboush, K. L., & Alyan, H. (2016). School psychology: Enhancing school climate and school connectedness. In M. M. Amer & G. H. Awad (Eds.), *Handbook of Arab American psychology* (pp. 318–330). New York: Routledge.

Hakim-Larson, J., & Menna, R. (2016). Acculturation and enculturation: Ethnic identity socialization process. In M. M. Amer & G. H. Awad (Eds.), *Handbook of Arab American psychology* (pp. 34–47). New York: Routledge.

Harb, C. (2016). The Arab region. In M. M. Amer & G. H. Awad (Eds.), *Handbook of Arab American psychology* (pp. 3–18). New York: Routledge.

Harper, B., & Tuckman, B. (2006). Racial identity beliefs and academic achievement: Does being black hold students back? *Social Psychology of Education, 9*, 381–403. https://doi.org/10.1007/s11218-006-9001-z.

Harter, S. (1999). *The construction of the self: A developmental perspective*. New York: Guilford Press.

Ibish, H. E. (2001). *Report on hate crimes and discrimination against Arab Americans 1998-2000*. Washington, DC: American Arab Anti-Discrimination Committee Research Institute.

Kenny, M. C., & McEachern, A. (2009). Children's self-concept: A multicultural comparison. *Professional School Counseling, 12*, 207–212. https://doi.org/10.5330/PSC.n.2010-12.207.

Moradi, B., & Hasan, N. T. (2004). Arab American persons' reported experiences of discrimination and mental health: The mediating role of personal control. *Journal of Counseling Psychology, 51*, 418–428. https://doi.org/10.1037/0022-0167.51.4.418.

Mossakowski, K. N. (2003). Coping with perceived discrimination: Does ethnic identity protect mental health? *Journal of Health and Social Behavior, 44*, 318–331. Retrieved from http://www.jstor.org/stable/1519782?origin=JSTOR-pdf

Read, J. G. (2008). Discrimination and identity formation in post 9/11 era: A comparison of Muslim and Christian Arab Americans. In A. Jamal & N. Naber (Eds.), *Race and Arab Americans before and after 9/11: From invisible citizens to visible subjects* (pp. 305–317). Syracuse, NY: Syracuse University Press.

Rivas-Drake, D., Hughes, D., & Way, N. (2008). A closer look at peer discrimination, ethnic identity, and psychological well-being among urban Chinese American sixth graders. *Journal of Youth and Adolescence, 37*, 12–21. https://doi.org/10.1007/s10964-007-9227-x.

Suleiman, M. F. (2000). *Teaching about Arab Americans: What social studies teachers should know*. Retrieved from http://eric.ed.gov/?id=ED442714

Twenge, J., & Crocker, J. (2002). Race and self-esteem: Meta-analyses comparing Whites, Blacks, Hispanics, Asians, and American Indians and comment on Gray-Little and Hafdahl (2000). *Psychological Bulletin, 128*, 371–408. https://doi.org/10.1037/0033-2909.128.3.371.

Wingfield, M., & Karaman, B. (2009). *Arab stereotypes and American educators*. Retrieved June 10, 2019, from https://www.adc.org/arab-stereotypes-and-american-educators/

Worrell, F. (2007). Ethnic identity, academic achievement, and global self-concept in four groups of academically talented adolescents. *Gifted Child Quarterly, 51*(1), 23–38. https://doi.org/10.1177/0016986206296655.

Wray-Lake, L., Syvertsen, A. K., & Flanagan, C. A. (2008). Contested citizenship and social exclusion: Adolescent Arab American immigrants' views of the social contract. *Applied Developmental Science, 12*, 84–92. https://doi.org/10.1080/10888690801997085.

Arab American Youth and Historical Contributors of Discrimination

Introduction

Since their immigration to the United States, Arabs in America have experienced stereotyping and discrimination, especially through the mainstream media and American government policies. As a result, this group, including Arab youth, has experienced racial complexities, cultural stereotypes, and identity issues in the United States. This chapter discusses the inconsistencies with racial categorization and identification by the American government, which has led to confusion with self-identification in the Arab community. Such confusion for Arab youth may leave them with a sense of lack of belonging and questions such as, "Who am I?" This stems from the fact that the American government has historically classified Arab Americans under ethnic and racial categories that do not necessarily correspond with how they identify themselves. This chapter presents the research regarding this issue and what has been found in various Arab communities. The majority of the research focuses on Arab adults in America. Nevertheless, the evidence may help us understand the experiences of Arab youth.

Through cultural conditioning, individuals acquire attitudes and values prevalent in society, which then leads to socializing according to their surroundings and current cultural values. Cultural conditioning leads to misconceptions and stereotypes which manifest in acts of discrimination. In the case of Arab culture, the process of cultural conditioning has been evident beginning with their immigration to the United States. Furthermore, researchers propose that cultural conditioning is a major factor in the way Arabs have been perceived in America. Therefore, this chapter presents a dialogue regarding the various misconceptions and negative cultural stereotypes that have been historically conditioned in the minds of the mainstream public through various forms of corporate media and enforced by government policies. Overall, the chapter serves to illustrate how discrimination against Arab Americans began and evolved as well as the governmental and societal factors that

R. Tabbah, *Arab American Youth*, Advancing Responsible Adolescent Development, https://doi.org/10.1007/978-3-030-66804-4_2

have contributed to misconceptions and stereotypes leading to discrimination against this ethnic group.

History of Immigration, Official Race Categorization, and Racial Identity

Arab Americans are a diverse group of individuals who come from 22 different Arabic-speaking countries in the Middle East and Northern Africa including Algeria, Bahrain, Comoros, Djibouti, Egypt, Iraq, Jordan, Kuwait, Lebanon, Libya, Mauritania, Morocco, Oman, Palestine, Qatar, Saudi Arabia, Somalia, Sudan, Syria, Tunisia, United Arab Emirates, and Yemen (Palacios & Trivedi, 2009). According to the Arab American Institute (AAI), the Arab American population is as diverse as their countries of origin with unique immigration experiences that have shaped their ethnic identity in the United States (AAI, n.d.). They come from multiple religious backgrounds, including—but not limited—to Judaism, Christianity, and Islam. Contrary to common belief, the majority of Arab Americans are of the Christian faith with approximately 35% being Roman or Eastern Catholic, 18% Eastern Orthodox, and 10% Protestant (AAI, 2003). Only about 24% of the Arab American population is of the Islamic faith, and 13% are identified as "Other religion/No affiliation" (AAI, 2003). The majority of Arab American descendants come from the first immigration wave of mostly Christian Arab immigrants; yet, Arab American Muslims currently represent the fastest growing sector of the Arab American community (AAI, n.d.).

Naber (2008) suggested that religious, ethnic, and linguistic diversity found within the Arab region contributes to the difficulties of the federal government and Arab communities finding a consensus on who is an Arab and what it means to be Arab. Joseph (1999) provided a compelling example of this diversity:

> There are Palestinians, Iraqis, Kuwaitis, Yemenis, Saudi Arabians, Bahreinis, Qataris, Duabis, Egyptians, Libyans, Tunisians, Moroccans, Algerians, Sudanese, Eritreans, and Mauritanians; there are Maronites, Catholics, Protestants, Greek Orthodox, Jews, Sunnis, Shi'a, Druze, Sufis, Alawites, Nestorians, Assyrians, Copts, Chaldeans, and Bahais; there are Berbers, Kurds, Armenians, bedu, gypsies, and many others with different languages, religions, ethnic, and national identifications and cultures who are all congealed as Arab in popular representation whether or not those people may identify as Arab. (p. 216)

This statement signifies the heterogeneity of this group, and how various factors such as nationality, religion, language, culture, and ethnicity may play crucial factors in identity formation. The statement also emphasizes the fact that just because an individual is from a known Arab region does not mean that they identify themselves as such. Further, it illustrates the diversity in religious practices and how not all Arabs are of the Islamic faith.

The literature discusses three significant waves of Arab immigration to America starting from over a century ago (Erickson & Al-Timimi, 2004) with each wave having significantly different experiences. While Arabs have been immigrating to the

United States prior to the nineteenth century, the first major group immigrated in the late 1880s (Naber, 2008). This first wave of immigration, occurring between the 1880s and World War I, consisted mostly of Christian merchants and farmers from the Greater Syria region. The majority of the population from this wave settled in Northeastern urban areas and Midwestern industrialized cities (Erickson & Al-Timimi, 2004). Researchers suggest that migrants from this group came to the United States due to economic necessity and for personal advancement (Naber, 2008). Starting with this initial wave, Arab identity has been disputed and shifted (Naber, 2008). According to researchers, this group was initially racially classified by the federal government as originating from "Turkey in Asia" (Samhan, 1999). Several years later in 1893, immigration reform classified Arabic-speaking immigrants as Syrians (Samhan, 1999). These terms established did not necessarily coincide with how individuals from this group identified (Naber, 2008). With the fall of the Ottoman Empire in 1917, the region was divided into separate countries referred to as the Arab World (Naber, 2008). This era contained another shift in identity definitions used by the federal government and Arab communities; for example, the national label "Lebanese" was politically legitimized and adopted by immigrants originating from Mount Lebanon in the 1920s (Naber, 2008; Naff, 1985).

In 1948, the year Israel was created, a second wave began including more professionals, Muslims, and displaced Palestinian refugees (Erickson & Al-Timimi, 2004). Naber (2008) indicated that this event was an impetus for the development of a sense of Arab nationalism in opposition to European colonialism and intervention in the Arab region in the decades to follow. Similar to the first wave of immigrant, the majority of this population also established themselves in Northeastern urban areas and Midwestern industrialized cities (Erickson & Al-Timimi, 2004).

The third wave began after the Arabs were defeated in the Arab–Israeli war in 1967. The majority demographic of this wave was Muslim; they settled in areas all over the United States. This wave of immigrants experienced a more negative reception and had more difficulty assimilating into mainstream society than did immigrants in the first two waves (Erickson & Al-Timimi, 2004). Researchers argue that this war instigated the emergence of a pan-ethnic Arab American identity due to the bias and pro-Israeli media reporting on the Middle East (Suleiman, 1999). This growing political and ethnic awareness was prompted by the derogatory racial overtones in the media toward the Arab (Awad, 1981).

While immigrants from the pre–World War II era came to the United States for economic and personal advancement, post–World War II immigrants majorly came to the United States after being displaced by factors such as war and colonialism (Naber, 2008). Post–World War II immigrants were also more diverse with immigrants coming from numerous Arab-speaking countries and including equal populations of Muslims and Christians (Suleiman, 1999). Naber (2008) reported that this group included Arabs from the Gulf region and North Africa with a greater population of Muslims, which provided an increased variation in appearance, skin color, cultural norms, and religious groups.

According to Naber (2008), relative to immigration policy, numerous, ever-changing terms historically used to categorize immigrants from Arabic-speaking countries have made racial classification of Arab immigrants in the United States extremely complex and contradictory. For example, as stated earlier, Arab immigrants in the 1880s were initially racially classified by the federal government as Turkish (Samhan, 1999). Subsequently, after immigration reform in 1893, Arabic-speaking immigrants were racially classified as Syrians (Samhan, 1999). Relatively more recently, in 1978, the federal government classified Arabs under "persons originating in Europe, the Middle East, and North Africa" (Samhan, 1999). About two decades later in 1997, Arab American community organizations in collaboration with the Office of Management and Budget identified a lack of consensus regarding the definition of an Arab ethnic category and called for research to improve the data on this population (Naber, 2008). To this date, no consensus has been reached regarding this definition.

The inconsistencies with government racial categorization can be seen in the various court cases throughout history described by researchers (Naber, 2008). Outlined by Naber (2008), these cases largely involved rights to United States citizenship based on the petitioners' race. In one case in Georgia in 1909 following the first significant wave of immigration, a Syrian named Costa George Najour was granted the right to citizenship based on the determination that he was considered to belong to the white race (Hassan, 2002). Conversely, a South Carolina case in 1914 denied George Dow, a Syrian immigrant, a petition to become a United States citizen (Samhan, 1999). This decision was based on the determination that Dow was not considered white, rather the judge considered him "Asiatic" (Naber, 2008). Often, religious identity was used to constitute the whiteness of Arabs; Christians were more likely to be identified as white than were their Muslim counterparts (Naber, 2008). While the Dow case was eventually appealed after it was determined that Syrians were part of a Semitic branch of the Caucasian race, this standard was never actively put into practice in future court cases (Hassan, 2002; Naber, 2008). For example, a Syrian was refused citizenship by the Supreme Court in 1923 based on the 1917 restrictive immigration act, which banned immigration from most countries in the east of the Persian Gulf (Naber, 2008). Subsequently, it was determined that Syrians do not fit within these restrictions (Samhan, 1999). These court case examples provide some insight on the racial complexities Arabs in America have experienced historically. The outcomes illustrate how, when it comes to race, some Arab Americans have passed as white, while others have not had the same privilege of passing as such, and others have self-identified according to explicit non-white racial and ethnic categories (Naber, 2008).

Cainkar (2008) stated that the racial formation processes in the United States have downgraded the social status of Arabs. The author argues that degradation is evident in public policies; mainstream representations; in social patterns of discrimination, separation, and exclusion; and in self-identification (Cainkar, 2008). Their experiences in the United States with racial identification throughout history likely leads to inconsistencies in how Arab Americans identify themselves. According to Cainkar (2008), some Arabs may identify themselves as white while others may not. Further, there may be some inconsistencies within Arab American communities regarding their political preferences and understanding of race

(Cainkar, 2008). Even though Arab Americans may have several options when it comes to race (e.g., white versus not white), these options do not negate the fact that they are a stigmatized group (Cainkar, 2008). Regardless of being stigmatized, Samhan (1999) posited that they are considered officially white by the federal government and ineligible for affirmative action. According to Cainkar (2008), Arabs hold a double burden: they are simultaneously excluded from being white and from being recognized as people of color by mainstream America. Wingfield (2006) further described the Arab American racial situation as an anomaly: "They are an officially 'white' ethnic group from the Third World, a large part of which is assimilated and/or affluent and highly educated. Yet they are widely perceived as culturally alien, may be treated as Other if not Enemy, and are vulnerable to discrimination and violence" (p. 255).

When it comes to race, Arab Americans do not generally share some of the traits that make other ethnic groups more visible. According to Suleiman (2000), they are less "racially visible" than other minorities such as Asian or African Americans (p. 6). This trait allows them to "blend in" with the European American population, meanwhile preserving their idiosyncratic cultural traits. Although they may be less identifiable physically, Arab Americans share other characteristics with other ethnic minority groups.

Schaefer (1990) discussed five characteristics or properties that differentiate ethnic minority groups from majority or dominant groups including visible physical or cultural characteristics, involuntary membership, in-group marriage, awareness of subordination, unequal treatment, and experience of prejudice. As an ethnic group, Arab Americans share with other ethnic groups all of these characteristics except for visible physical characteristics (Suleiman, 2000). Suleiman (2000) suggested that the most remarkable characteristic of Arab Americans as a group that is invisible is their unequal treatment and experiences of prejudice and discrimination. Regardless of their invisibility as an ethnic minority group and their labeling as a "white" ethnic group, they have experienced as much discrimination and prejudice as other racially visible minority groups (Suleiman, 2000).

Saloom (2005) examined the issues of race with Arab Americans. The author claimed that there is much confusion in the examination of race and Arab Americans and that this confusion is exacerbated by interchanging the terms of Arab and Muslim. The fact that Arab Americans are officially classified as white is highly problematic (Saloom, 2005). The reason being that, essentially, Arabs are considered white, until a crisis happens and then they are not. Saloom (2005) explained:

> Some scholars contend that Arab-Americans are only considered white in an "honorary" sense and that whenever a relevant national crisis occurs that "honorary" status is revoked. This honorary white status is highly problematic because Arab-Americans are thereby whitewashed, and claims of racism and discrimination are not taken seriously. (p. 59)

The discrimination and prejudice that Arab Americans faced after 9/11 especially demonstrated that Arab Americans, while considered white by the United States government, were non-whites, were anything but white, and were considered the "other" (Saloom, 2005).

Based on the history of racial categorization, establishing a true census of the Arab American population is almost impossible. At the time of the 2000 United States Census, an ancestry question was incorporated into the long version of the form (Abdulrahim, 2008). Estimates obtained from this ancestry question on the 2000 United States Census placed the Arab American population at about 1.25 million (Samhan, 2007). The problem inherent in this is that the census defines people who trace their origins to the Middle East and North Africa as white. Therefore, information on how persons of Arab ancestry respond to the race question are non-existent (Abdulrahim, 2008), and the estimated population from the United States is grossly under representative. Individuals who mark the "some other race" category and write Arab are automatically entered as white, which undermines their self-identification as non-white and negates the data on percentages of Arab Americans who identified themselves as "white" and who conversely identified themselves as "other race—Arab" (Abdulrahim, 2008).

The most recent 2010 United States Census placed the Arab American population at about 1.5 million (Asi & Beaulieu, 2013). The Arab American Institute (AAI) reported that this was about a 72% growth from the 2000 United States Census (AAI, 2014). According to the AAI (2014), the number of Americans claiming Arab ancestry has more than doubled since 1980 when the United States Census originally began measuring ethnic origins, which makes this group the largest growing Arab diaspora group in the world. The majority of the Arab American population per the Census consists of Lebanese (485,917), Egyptian (179,853), Syrian (147,426), Palestinian (83,241), Moroccan (74,908), Iraqi (73,896), Jordanian (60,056), and Yemeni (29,358) (Asi & Beaulieu, 2013).

In contrast to the 2010 United States Census, the Arab American Institute Foundation (AAI, 2014) reported an adjusted number of over 3.6 million, which leaves about half of the population unaccounted for by the Census. According to demographics reported by the AAI, Arab Americans reside all over the nation. However, up to 94% live in metropolitan areas with the top five being Los Angeles, Detroit, New York, Chicago, and Washington DC (AAI, 2014). The majority live in ten states: California, Michigan, New York, Texas, Florida, Illinois, New Jersey, Ohio, Massachusetts, and Pennsylvania (AAI, n.d.). The AAI provides reports on the most current Arab demographics in the United States (AAI, n.d.). California has an estimated population of 817,455 Arab Americans with the majority residing in Los Angeles County. Michigan's estimated population is greater than 500,000 with the majority in Wayne County. At number 3, New York has 449,187 estimated Arab Americans with the majority residing in Kings County. At number 4, Texas estimates around 274,701 Arab Americans with the majority in Dallas County. Florida is estimated at 301,881 with the majority living in Miami-Dade County. Illinois estimates at 256,395 with the majority in Cook County. New Jersey's estimated population is 257,868, the majority in Hudson and Bergen Counties. Ohio ranks eight with an estimated population of 197,439 with the majority residing in Cuyahoga County. Massachusetts and Pennsylvania estimate at 195,450 and 182,610 with majorities in Middlesex and Philadelphia Counties, respectively.

Shryock (2008) discussed the racialization of Arabs and Muslims in the United States following 9/11. The author emphasized how the United States government imposes the white identification on Arabs even though they may not necessarily identify themselves with this category. The Detroit Arab American Study (DAAS) was conducted in 2003 with a sample of 1016 participants in Wayne, Macomb, and Oakland counties of Michigan in order to understand Arab perspective on race, identity, and ancestry (Shryock, 2008). The following three questions regarding racial and ethnic identification were asked: (1) Do you feel the term "Arab American" describes you? (2) Is there any other term like "Arab American" that better describes you? and (3) What is your race? (Check all that apply): (1) White; (2) Black, African American, or Negro; (3) American Indian or Alaska Native; (4) Asian; (5) Pacific Islander; (6) Other (Specify). The researchers reportedly coded answers differently than the United States Census in that write-in responses of "Arab," "Lebanese," and "Palestinian" were not recoded as "white" when respondents did not check the "white" category.

Results showed that 70% of the participants were willing to identify themselves as "Arab American," whereas 30% preferred to be called something else. Participants offered approximately 100 different identities when asked if there was another term that better describes them, including "just American," "Iraqi," "Egyptian Christian," "Arabic," "Lebanese American," "American Lebanese," and other versions of national, regional, and religious labels (Shryock, 2008). Further, none of the participants preferred to use an existent racial alternative, including white, black, Asian, or even "of color" (p. 89). The author also noted that Christians were less likely than Muslims to accept the label "Arab American."

In terms of the third question regarding race, 64% who identified themselves as "white" were more likely to be Christian and live in the middle- and upper-middle-class suburbs, where they intermingled with a white majority. Conversely, the 31% who identified themselves as "other" were more likely to live in heavily concentrated Muslim enclaves of Dearborn, Dearborn Heights, and adjacent neighborhoods in Detroit (Shryock, 2008). Further, 73% of the Christian sample identified themselves as white, while only 50% of the Muslim population identified themselves the same. Participants who were born in America and those with United States citizenship were more likely to identify themselves as white than non-citizens and those born abroad. Additionally, participants who reported that they do not self-identify with the "Arab American" label were also more likely to identify themselves as white.

Cainkar (2008) conducted a study with 102 Arab Muslims in Chicago to examine their views of racial structures in the United States. Forty-five percent were female. The majority of the sample was middle class (62%) while 18% were low income and 20% upper middle class and wealthy. Ages ranged from 19 to over 50 years. Education levels included high school or less (14%), some college or BS/BA (43%), and postgraduate (42%). Twenty-nine percent were born in the United States. Participants were asked the question: "There have been discussions about whether Arabs are white or not, with different points of view. Do you think Arabs are white, not white, or what?"

Results showed that 63% of the respondents responded that Arabs were not white, 20% said they were white, and the final 17% provided ambiguous responses. Participants who said Arabs were not white made this choice based on the following factors: their treatment in the American society, skin color and other phenotypic criteria, the fact that Arabs are multiracial, cultural and historical difference they hold from Europeans, and Arab distinctiveness. The author reported that the majority of participants who said Arabs were white immediately used examples of government forms, such as the United States Census, job and school application forms. Results showed that Arabs acknowledge that they are to check the "white" category on forms; the majority say they do, even though they do not agree that Arabs are white (Cainkar, 2008). The author discussed various responses based on the themes that arose. Thirty six percent of respondents claimed Arabs were not white based on the way Arabs are treated in American society. The majority were American born. The respondents noted the Arab experience with political exclusion and discriminatory treatment in schools and in the public domain. One participant stated:

> Arabs are definitely not white. That categorization comes from the treatment of a community by the institutions of American society. Arabs in the schools face the same institutional racism as other students of color. (Chicago-born male) (p. 63)

Twenty-eight percent of respondents stated that Arabs were not white because of their skin color and other phenotypic criteria, such as facial features and types of hair (Cainkar, 2008). For example, one Kuwaiti-born female expressed:

> We are definitely not white. But the whole idea of color makes no sense to me. My neighbor is black according to the census forms but she is lighter than I am. There are Arabs that are lighter than white people. I don't think people should be classified like that, by color. I don't agree with it at all. If I was to classify myself, I would consider myself brown. I would not consider myself white. My youngest and oldest child would be white and my middle child brown. It does not work for me. (p. 66)

Another United States-born female stated:

> People look at me and they don't know what I am. They know I am not white or black. People think I am Hispanic. Brown is in the middle. (p. 65)

Twenty four percent of the participants entailed the third most common response of Arabs not being white because Arabs cannot be a racial group due to the Arab world encompassing various geographic regions and skin colors (Cainkar, 2008). One United States-born female respondent stated:

> I think Arabs should have a different category until things change…If you look on the map, Arab countries cover two continents, and the white-white and dark black. If this is my cousin and he's dark, and he's from Africa, are you going to call him white? (p. 66)

The fourth theme found among 20% of the respondents was that Arabs were not white because their culture and heritage is different from Caucasian/European (Cainkar, 2008). These respondents reportedly felt that they were allowing their own Arab heritage and culture to be encompassed into that of Europe. A United States-born female participant expressed:

> Their history and culture is quite separate from Europe's. I find it a disgrace that the Arab people should be so blatantly insulted by the disregard of their history. (p. 67)

Finally, 17% of the participants provided ambiguous responses to the race question, demonstrating the difficulties they have with the idea of race and Arabs being forced into one racial category. An example statement from a Chicago-born female is as follows:

> I don't really know. I think for me, it's always been white because of what I look like. I consider myself white. That's probably a personal reflection because my skin color is white. I've always thought all Arabs were white. I've never really thought of them as being non-white. But, again, why do we say we're white, because we're not white. Like people say, "you put 'white,'" and I think that it just doesn't make sense. I don't know what white means in terms of technical definition. Is it people who live north of the equator? I don't know how the experts have defined it. If you ask anybody, they say to put white as a race. Do I think we're white? I don't think so. (p. 68)

There is a lack of research on Arab American adolescents' views of being labeled under the "white" designation. In one study regarding this issue, Ajrouch (2004) found that the Arab American adolescents in this study distinguished themselves from white America, regardless of them being labeled as white by the government. The Arab American girls in this study further distinguished themselves from white girls, which possibly speaks to the role of gender in racial identity formation for Arab American adolescent girls.

In conclusion, the racial classification system in the United States regarding individuals descending from the Arab world has led to great confusion and inconsistencies between and within the Arab community when it comes to self-identification. The disparities are seen in the research discussed above. For example, comparatively speaking, the majority of the DAAS study sample in Detroit, Michigan said Arabs were white (64%), while 31% said they were non-white (Shryock, 2008). Conversely, in the study by Cainkar (2008) in Chicago, 63% of the sample reported that Arabs were not white, 20% reported that Arabs were white, and the remaining sample gave ambiguous responses. Cainkar (2016) suggests that Arab Americans have been socialized to check the white box on government forms because they are officially categorized as such, and there is no "Arab" option to choose otherwise. As the research shows, they do this whether they agree with the categorization or not (Cainkar, 2016). This type of confusion may interplay with how these individuals perceive discrimination and are affected by such experiences. For example, Abdulrahim, James, Yamout, and Baker (2012) found that Muslims, those with darker skin, and individuals who identified themselves as non-white reported more discrimination than those who were non-Muslim, had lighter skin, and identified themselves as white. Further, some Arabs may identify themselves as and/or pass as white, while others do not necessarily hold this privilege because of obvious phenotypic characteristics that identify them as non-white (Awad & Amayreh, 2016). The inconsistencies in the classification system has also contributed to the various and disparate outcomes of government policies and civil liberties pertaining to this ethnic group; while in some cases they were considered white, in others they were categorized as non-white and their rights were infringed upon. Furthermore, the manner in which Arab cultures are perceived by the mainstream public may have an impact on how Arabs are treated by the majority.

Cultural Stereotypes: Effects of Cultural Conditioning

Cultural conditioning refers to the process by which people acquire attitudes and values that are passed on by society (Henderson, 1988), and the process in which people socialize according to their surroundings and current cultural values (Lim & Ang, 2008). This process affects the way people think about and act, react, and behave toward other people. Cultural conditioning is taught through families, government, media, schools, and other surroundings. It is required to integrate or assimilate successfully with society; however, cultural conditioning hinders society and allows them to follow blindly (Henderson, 1988). This is especially true in the case of the American society in the portrayal of Arab American cultures (Suleiman, 2000).

Suleiman (2000) discussed the effects of cultural conditioning on Arabs in America. There are various factors that contribute to cultural conditioning that affects how society views minorities (Suleiman, 2000). In the case of Arabs, the mass media plays a significant role in shaping the attitudes of individuals and groups toward Arab cultures by enhancing stereotypes (Suleiman, 2000). Research indicates that—even prior to 9/11—the media has forced Arabs into a world of stereotyping and discrimination (e.g., Banks, 2009; Nieto, 1996).

The school system further perpetuates stereotypes and discrimination through lack of representation or misrepresentation of Arab cultures (Nieto, 1996). In the education realm, Arab Americans are rarely included in the multicultural paradigm. The majority of multicultural educators' books, articles, and programs do not include them. More frequently included in this paradigm are the racial categories of white, African American, Hispanic or Latino, Asian Pacific, and Native American. The lack of representation of the Arab culture in schools and the field of education leads to more misunderstanding and less tolerance of the culture. Furthermore, because Arab Americans are lumped with the European American or "white" category, they are highly underrepresented and made culturally and racially invisible. Curriculum reform regarding Arab cultures has been called on by researchers for decades prior to the terrorist attacks of 9/11 (e.g., Al-Qazzaz, Afifi, & Shabbas, 1978). Despite these efforts, there has been a serious lack of effort to acknowledge Arab cultures in education systems in the United States (Starr, 1990), at least up until 9/11.

Through the process of cultural conditioning, Arab cultures have historically been misrepresented by American media and various other sources. A common misconception is that all Arabs are of the Muslim faith, all Muslims are Arabs, and the two terms are interchangeable (Al-Hazza & Lucking, 2005). Although the Islamic and Arab cultures are very similar in many ways, these terms are in no way interchangeable. The misconception disregards the other religious groups of this ethnicity, including, but not limited to, those of the Christian and Jewish faith. In fact, only

20% of the world's population of Muslims are Arab (Suleiman, 2000). Naber (2008) listed the top six countries with the largest Muslim population, none of which are considered Arab, as: Indonesia, Pakistan, Bangladesh, India, Turkey, and Iran.

Negative images of Arab American people and their culture in the media have permeated American society (Suleiman, 2000). Generally, the most contact that American society has with Arabs and information they receive about their countries and culture is through the media (Suleiman, 1996). Anderson (1991) argued that the US media has certainly done their part when it comes to anti-Arab propaganda and encouraging Arab-bashing. The majority of what the American public sees in the media about Arab people and their culture is negative, and because they generally have no other contact with Arabs to contradict images in the media, the negative images usually prevail (M.F. Suleiman, 2000). Researchers suggest that the way Arab immigrants have been received and treated throughout history is related to the manner in which they have been portrayed and perceived through mainstream media and the public (Naber, 2008). Consequently, these negative perceptions and portrayals have led to prejudice and discrimination against Arabs in America prior to and especially after the 9/11 terrorist attacks. Following 9/11, negative stereotypes and perceptions regarding Arab cultures and communities gained even more momentum and resulted in a significant increase in discrimination against Arab American individuals and communities. Arabs, and those perceived to be Arab, were generally blamed for the attacks and targeted by the mainstream media and public.

Conclusion

Beginning with their immigration to the United States, Arab Americans have faced various forms of discrimination. This chapter provided a background of factors contributing to discrimination of Arab Americans throughout history, which are crucial in understanding their experiences in the United States. This chapter illustrated how factors of government racial identification systems have contributed to discrimination and how this system has also led to conflict in identity formation for Arab Americans. The inconsistencies of racial classification throughout history for individuals of Arab descent have further convoluted matters. While the research available largely focused on adults, we expect the evidence to translate to Arab youth as well. One study demonstrated that, indeed, the Arab youth in the study differentiated themselves from the white racial classification. More studies need to be conducted to explore this phenomenon. Further complicating identity development, racial classification in the school systems leads to a significant lack of representation of Arab youth.

The cultural conditioning of mainstream society's perceptions has further contributed to the discrimination experiences of this group. The misconceptions engrained through the mass media and other sources have culturally conditioned majority of the society with negative perceptions regarding Arab and Arab American cultures. Of significance, this process is manifested in the American school systems with the lack of representation and/or misrepresentation of Arab cultures in multicultural curricula, which, researchers suggest, is in and of itself a form of discrimination. When the school environment is as such, Arab youth become at-risk for developmental complications.

References

AAI. (2003). *Arab Americans*. Retrieved February 20, 2019, from http://www.aaiusa.org/arab-americans/22/demographics

AAI. (2014). *Demographics*. Retrieved November 17, 2018, from https://d3n8a8pro7vhmx.cloudfront.net/aai/pages/9843/attachments/original/1460668240/National_Demographic_Profile_2014.pdf?1460668240

AAI. (n.d.). *Demographics*. Retrieved September 23, 2019, from http://www.aaiusa.org/demographics

Abdulrahim, S. (2008). "Whiteness" and the Arab immigrant experience. In A. Jamal & N. Naber (Eds.), *Race and Arab Americans before and after 9/11*. Syracuse, NY: Syracuse University Press.

Abdulrahim, S., James, S. A., Yamout, R., & Baker, W. (2012). Discrimination and psychological distress: Does whiteness matter for Arab Americans? *Social Science & Medicine, 75*(12), 2116–2123. https://doi.org/10.1016/j.socscimed.2012.07.030.

Ajrouch, K. J. (2004). Gender, race, and symbolic boundaries: Contested spaces of identity among Arab American adolescents. *Sociological Perspectives, 47*(4), 371–391.

Al-Hazza, T., & Lucking, B. (2005). The minority of suspicion: Arab Americans. *MultiCultural Review, 14*, 32–38.

Al-Qazzaz, A., Afifi, R., & Shabbas, A. (1978). *The Arab world: A handbook for teachers*. Berkeley, CA: NAJDA (Women Concerned about the Middle East).

Anderson, J. (1991). Blame the Arabs: Tensions in the Gulf bring bigotry at home. *The Progressive, 55*(2), 28–29.

Asi, M., & Beaulieu, D. (2013). *Arab households in the United States: 2006–2010*. Retrieved September 10, 2019, from https://www.census.gov/library/publications/2013/acs/acsbr10-20.html

Awad, G. (1981). The Arab Americans: An invisible minority awakens. *News Circle*, pp. 31–32.

Awad, G. H., & Amayreh, W. M. (2016). Discrimination: Heightened prejudice post 9/11 and psychological outcomes. In M. M. Amer & G. H. Awad (Eds.), *Handbook of Arab American psychology* (pp. 63–75). New York: Routledge.

Banks, J. A. (2009). *Teaching strategies for ethnic studies* (8th ed.). Boston, MA: Allyn and Bacon.

Cainkar, L. (2008). Thinking outside the box: Arabs and race in the United States. In A. Jamal & N. Naber (Eds.), *Race and Arab Americans before and after 9/11: From invisible citizens to visible subjects* (pp. 46–80). Syracuse, NY: Syracuse University Press.

Cainkar, L. (2016). Race and racialization: Demographic trends and the process of reckoning social place. In M. M. Amer & G. H. Awad (Eds.), *Handbook of Arab American psychology* (pp. 19–33). New York: Routledge.

Erickson, C. D., & Al-Timimi, N. R. (2004). *Counseling and psychotherapy with Arab American clients*. Boston, MA: Allyn and Bacon.

Hassan, S. (2002). Arabs, race and the post-September 11 National Security State. *Middle East Report, 224*, 16. https://doi.org/10.2307/1559418.

Henderson, J. L. (1988). The cultural unconscious. *Quadrant, 21*(2), 7–16.

Joseph, S. (1999). Against the grain of the nation- The Arab. In M. W. Suleiman (Ed.), *Arabs in America: Building a new future* (pp. 257–272). Philadelphia, PA: Temple University Press.

Lim, E. A. C., & Ang, S. H. (2008). Hedonic vs. utilitarian consumption: A cross-cultural perspective based on cultural conditioning. *Journal of Business Research, 61*, 225–232. https://doi.org/10.1016/j.jbusres.2007.06.004.

Naber, N. (2008). Introduction: Arab Americans and U.S. racial formations. In A. Jamal & N. Naber (Eds.), *Race and Arab Americans before and after 9/11* (pp. 1–45). Syracuse, NY: Syracuse University Press.

Naff, A. (1985). *Becoming American: The Early Arab immigrant experience*. Carbondale, IL: Southern Illinois University Press.

Nieto, S. (1996). *Affirming diversity: The sociopolitical context of multicultural education* (2nd ed.). New York: Longman.

Palacios, E. D., & Trivedi, P. (2009). Increasing cultural literacy: Historical perspectives and cultural characteristics of minority groups. In J. M. Jones (Ed.), *The psychology of multiculturalism in the schools: A primer for practice, training, and research*. National Association of School Psychology: Bethesda, MD.

Saloom, R. (2005). I know you are, but what am I? Arab-American experiences through the critical race theory lens. *Hamline Journal of Public Law & Policy, 27*, 55–76.

Samhan, H. H. (1999). Not quite white: Race classification and the Arab-American experience. In M. Suleiman (Ed.), *Arabs in America: Building a new future* (pp. 209–226). Philadelphia, PA: Temple University Press.

Samhan, H. H. (2007). *By the numbers. Comprehensive report on Arab American community demographics*. Retrieved July 21, 2009, from http://www.allied-media.com/Arab-American/Arab_demographics.htm

Schaefer, R. T. (1990). *Racial and ethnic groups*. Glenview, IL: Scott Foresman.

Shryock, A. (2008). The moral analogies of race: Arab American identity, color politics, and the limits of racialized citizenship. In A. Jamal & N. Naber (Eds.), *Race and Arab Americans before and after 9/11*. Syracuse, NY: Syracuse University Press.

Starr, S. F. (1990). Colleges can help America overcome its ignorance of Arab language and culture. *The Chronicle of Higher Education*, p. B2.

Suleiman, M. F. (1996, November 6–10). *Educating the Arab American child: Implications for teachers*. Paper presented at the National Association for Multicultural Education, St. Paul, MN.

Suleiman, M. F. (2000). *Teaching about Arab Americans: What Social Studies Teachers Should Know*. Retrieved from http://eric.ed.gov/?id=ED442714

Suleiman, M. W. (1999). Introduction: The Arab American experience. In M. W. Suleiman (Ed.), *Arabs in America: Building a new future* (pp. 1–21). Philadelphia, PA: Temple University Press.

Wingfield, M. (2006). Arab Americans: Into the multicultural mainstream. *Equity & Excellence in Education, 39*, 253–266. https://doi.org/10.1080/10665680600788453.

Arab American Youth and Discrimination in the Pre-9/11 Era

Introduction

Arabs in America have long experienced discrimination. While common belief holds that the terrorist attacks of 9/11 were catalyst to discrimination against Arabs in the United States, the evidence shows otherwise. This chapter details the types of discrimination experienced by Arabs in America in the pre-9/11 era. The dialogue illustrates that 9/11 was not the starting point of discrimination for Arabs. Rather, the event was a turning point, as researchers have suggested. Discrimination prior to 9/11 was evident in multiple facets of society including governmental policy, mainstream media, and even the school system. The narrative demonstrates how deeply rooted stereotypes and discrimination are for this ethnic group, including the American education system.

Discrimination Against Arabs in the Pre-9/11 Era

Similar to other ethnic groups in the United States, Arab Americans have faced a long history of racism and discrimination (Saloom, 2005). Because attention to Arab Americans was magnified by the media, government, and general public after the terrorist attacks of 9/11 (Saloom, 2005), some may be led to believe that this event caused the misconceptions and discrimination toward this group. However, stereotyping, racism, and discrimination against this group can be traced back to the beginning of their immigration to the United States.

Arab Americans were often denied voting rights in the South (Saloom, 2005; Samhan, 1999). For example, a candidate for coroner in the 1920s in Birmingham, Alabama, distributed campaign flyers that stated: "They have disqualified the negro, an American citizen, from voting in the white primary. The Greek and Syrian should also be disqualified. I DON'T WANT THEIR VOTE. If I can't be elected by white

R. Tabbah, *Arab American Youth*, Advancing Responsible Adolescent Development, https://doi.org/10.1007/978-3-030-66804-4_3

men, I don't want the office" (Hitti, 1924, p. 89). The Ku Klux Klan targeted Arab Americans because they were often identified as people of color (Samhan, 1999). In the South during the 1950s, many Arabs were not allowed to use the same facilities as those designated as exclusively white (Shakir, 1997).

Common stereotypes of Arab Americans are perpetuated by the images that have been historically portrayed in the media, including villains and terrorists in films, in the pre-9/11 era. Movies such as *Siege, Delta Force, Patriot Games, Back to the Future,* and *True Lies* are exemplary of the portrayals of Arab Americans in Hollywood films (Wingfield, 2006). Rainey (2004) posited that such portrayals of the media keep circulating because it is easy for movie makers to use "Arabs" as villains or terrorists: "When writers want to portray a terrorist, or someone who is threatening, they put them in Middle Eastern attire, give them an accent, and make them look Arab. That's a stereotype used often because it's very quick and easy."

Research shows that Arabs have been stereotyped in the media as early as 1897 when Thomas Edison made a film in which "Arab" women wore provocative clothes while seductively dancing in front of a group of men (Al-Hazza & Lucking, 2005). This illustrates a long-held perception of women being subordinates of men in Arab culture. A prominent researcher in racial and ethnic studies, Jack Shaheen is known for his evaluation of the media and stereotypes portrayed regarding Arabs and Arab Americans. Through his research, there is compelling evidence that Arabs have been increasingly portrayed in the media as culturally backward, uncivilized, exotic, and potential enemies of the United States dating back to the 1970s (Shaheen, 2001). For example, there were images of rich oil sheikhs threatening the United States economy accompanying harems of women and belly dancers in 1970, cartoons depicting Palestinians as rats or fleas in the 1980s, and various movies in the 1980s and 1990s perpetuating the image of Arab terrorists (Naber, 2008).

Shaheen (1985) conducted a review of the images purported by various media sources in the United States. The author included images in television, motion pictures, and publishing industries. Television, in particular, may influence the minds of children, especially for children who have no personal experience with Arabs, and their sole knowledge comes from what is shown on television (Cortes, 1979; Shaheen, 1985). Shaheen (1985) cited examples of Saturday morning cartoon shows that feature stereotypical Arabs, including Ali Boo-Boo, Abdul-O, the Un-Cool-O, the Desert Rat, and the Sheik in Wolf's Clothing, where these characters "lurk in the shadows of pyramids and harm the innocent" (p. 164). Wrestling programs on television feature the so-called Arab wrestlers—the Iron Sheik, Akbar the Great, and Abdullah the Butchers—who "wrestle for the sheer pleasure of inflicting pain on others" (p. 164). In television comedies, Arabs were depicted as having too much money and too many wives, and inaccurate portrayals of Arab customs have been learned through shows such as *Alice* and *CHiPs* (Shaheen, 1985). Images in motion pictures in the 1980s showed Arabs as serious threats to the world (e.g., *Network, The Formula, Rollover, Wrong Is Right*), sexually depraved (e.g., *Bolero, Protocol, Sahara*), and less than human (e.g., *Time After Time, Things Are Tough All Over, Best Defense*) (Shaheen, 1985). In publications, Arabs have been depicted as religious fanatics, warmongers, and inept assassins determined to destroy Israel and the

West with nuclear weapons (e.g., *The Haj, Key to Rebecca, Evergreen*) (Shaheen, 1985). In addition, the 1978 version of the Merriam-Webster Thesaurus (Merriam-Webster, 1978) cited synonyms for "Arab" as "vagabond," "peddler," "bum," "derelict," and "tramp" (Shaheen, 1985, p. 165).

Saloom (2005) further discussed the racial phenomenon of Arab Americans being invisible and hyper-visible at the same time. The author offered an excerpt by Kadi (1994) that illustrates this phenomenon:

> As Arabs, like other people of color in this racist society, our race is simultaneously emphasized and ignored. For long periods of time no one can remember that Arabs even exist...Of course, this forgetfulness changes once there is another 'crisis' in the Middle East...During crisis, Arabs can be reassured we exist as a distinct racial group. We will remember it, in the dark of night and the light of day. We will feel the effects of the social construction of "the Arabs" that has cast us as enemy, other, fanatical terrorist, crazy Muslim. (p. xvi)

Abudabbeh (2005) discussed how certain events have contributed to an increased visibility of Arab Americans and how, essentially, Arabs are invisible until they are not. Several historical events—such as the discovery of oil in Arab countries, the creation of the State of Israel and the creation of a disenfranchised Palestinian refugee population, and the beginnings of the Islamization of the Arab world—served as catalysts to the visibility of Arab Americans (Abudabbeh, 2005). With such events, the average Americans became more aware of Arab Americans; however, this awareness was associated with negative stereotypes (Abudabbeh, 2005). This period was followed by a period where images seemed to change to less negative with figures, such as the entertainer Casey Kasem, cabinet member Donna Shallah, and comedian Danny Thomas, who were all highly assimilated early immigrants (Abudabbeh, 2005). Abudabbeh (2005) indicated that assimilation was easier for early immigrants who were Christians. Immigrants, such as Danny Thomas, proved to be essential in enabling reduction of negative stereotypes of Arabs with other recent immigrants in the United States (Abudabbeh, 2005). This period of improvement, however, was soon halted following the terrorist attacks of 9/11, and any positive images of Arab Americans were reverted back to historically negative stereotypes (Abudabbeh, 2005). Consequently, when they were easily assimilating with no related events catching attention of the mainstream public and media, Arab American images were less negative; hence, they were invisible. However, this changed with crises involving Arabs. In essence, these types of events cause Arabs to be "seen" by mainstream society, lead to the generalization of Arab Americans, and allow negative stereotypes to prevail.

Naber (2008) outlined the various experiences Arabs encountered in the post–World War II era up until the terrorist attacks of 9/11. Post–World War II marked an era of increased anti-Arab discourses and policies along with an increase in pan-ethnic Arab American political activism (Naber, 2008). The author used the term "anti-Arab racism" in order:

> to locate Arab American marginalization within the context of US histories of immigrant exclusion (e.g., the history of Asian exclusion, anti-Mexican racism, and Japanese internment) in which the racialization of particular immigrants as different than and inferior to

whites has relied upon culturalist and nationalist logics that assume "they" are intrinsically unassimilable and threatening to national security (Naber, 2008, p. 31).

Naber (2008) argued that experiences of racial exclusion for Arabs increase when there is some type of political crisis. The author described anti-Arab racism in the post–World War II era as being an interplay of the US involvement in the Middle East, anti-Arab media representations, and the institutionalization of government policies that explicitly target Arabs/Arab Americans in the United States (Naber, 2008). Naber (2008) discussed the coordination between historical shifts in the US involvement in the Middle East and shifts in media representations of "the Arab" (p. 37). For example, anti-Arab racism was exacerbated after the 1967 Arab–Israeli war: with the intensification of the US involvement in the Arab region came further negative media representations and anti-Arab discrimination and harassment in the United States (Naber, 2008). This era also marked a conflation of the terms "Arab" and "Muslim," where dialogues in the United States increasingly portrayed the assumption that all Arabs are Muslims and all Muslims are Arabs and that the religion of Islam is backward, uncivilized, and violently misogynistic toward women (Naber, 2008).

Next, Naber (2008) discussed the interplay between the US involvement in the Arab region and the establishment of government policy targeting explicitly Arabs in America. For example, Nixon's Operation Boulder in 1972 was one of the first FBI policies that targeted individuals of Arab descent by authorizing the FBI to harass individuals of Arab descent with phone calls and visits without evidence of criminal activity, based on the assumption that these individuals might have a relationship with terrorist activities in Palestine and Israel (Akram, 2002; Naber, 2008). Further, in 1978, the FBI director ran Operation Abscam and had agents pose as rich Arabs trying to bribe politicians and elected officials, essentially with the intention to create the impression that Arabs are a threat to politics in America (Naber, 2008). Additionally, there was a scenario in which the Department of Energy printed thousands of bumper stickers with the statement: "The Faster You Drive, The Richer They Get…Driving 75 is Sheik; Driving 55 is Chic" (p. 35). Then, in 1994, President Clinton's counterterrorism bill legitimized the targeting of Arabs in the United States by the federal government (Naber, 2008). This bill called for deportation of non-citizens without presenting evidence to the individuals involved, rather based on secret evidence only known by the government (Naber, 2008).

Stereotypes of Arabs in the education setting can also be dated back in research as early as the 1970s (Saloom, 2005). Jarrar (1983) examined textbooks in the 1970s and found that Arabs were "portrayed as primitive, backward, desert-dwelling, nomadic, war-loving, terroristic, and full of hate" (p. 388). Arabs in the multicultural curriculum have historically been nonexistent or misrepresented, which in and of itself is a form of discrimination (Wingfield, 2006). Researchers have called for curriculum reform regarding Arab and Arab American cultures for years prior to the terrorist attacks (e.g., Suleiman, 2000; Wingfield & Salam, 1993). Studies conducted after 9/11 have found that stereotypes continue to permeate both history and geography books with the focus being on camels, Bedouins, and deserts (Wingfield

& Karaman, 2009). Stereotypical images of Arabs taught at an early age to children allow negative stereotypes to be perpetuated in society and have detrimental effects on Arab American children's identity formation (Saloom, 2005).

Conclusion

The literature provides compelling evidence that discrimination across various societal facets against Arab Americans existed prior to 9/11 and as early as the 1800s when Arab immigrants began arriving in the United States. These range from negative media representations in the 1890s to negative portrayals in educational textbooks in the 1970s. Arab youth were not spared from the impact of such portrayals, since the research demonstrates how stereotypes and discrimination in the pre-9/11 era also infiltrated the education system. An analysis of images of Arabs in mainstream media since the 1800s indicates the longevity of the problem and how deeply rooted these stereotypes and misperceptions are in American society, including the education system.

References

Abudabbeh, N. (2005). Arab American families: Assessment and treatment. In E. P. Congress & M. J. González (Eds.), *Multicultural perspectives in working with families* (2nd ed., pp. 228–241). New York: Springer.

Akram, S. (2002). The aftermath of September 11, 2001: The targeting of Arabs and Muslims in America. *Arab Studies Quarterly, Spring*, 61–118.

Al-Hazza, T., & Lucking, B. (2005). The minority of suspicion: Arab Americans. *MultiCultural Review, 14*, 32–38.

Cortes, C. (1979). The societal curriculum and the school curriculum: Allies or antagonists? *Educational Leadership, 36*(7), 475–479. Retrieved from http://www.ascd.org/ASCD/pdf/journals/ed_lead/el_197904_cortes.pdf.

Hitti, P. K. (1924). *The Syrians in America, by Philip K. Hitti, with an introduction by Talcott Williams*. New York: George H. Doran Company.

Jarrar, S. A. (1983). The treatment of Arabs in U.S. social studies textbooks: Research findings and recommendations. In E. Ghareeb (Ed.), *Split vision: The portrayal of Arabs in the American media* (pp. 381–390). Washington, DC: American Arab Affairs Council.

Kadi, J. (1994). Introduction. In J. Kadi (Ed.), *Food for our grandmothers: Writings by Arab-American and Arab-Canadian Feminists* (pp. xiii–xx). Cambridge, MA: South End Press.

Merriam-Webster. (1978). *The Merriam-Webster thesaurus*. Springfield, MA: Merriam-Webster.

Naber, N. (2008). Introduction: Arab Americans and U.S. racial formations. In A. Jamal & N. Naber (Eds.), *Race and Arab Americans before and after 9/11* (pp. 1–45). Syracuse, NY: Syracuse University Press.

Rainey, D. (2004). *Media and image-building*. Retrieved January 26, 2010, from http://www.alhewar.com/rainey.html

Saloom, R. (2005). I know you are, but what am I? Arab-American experiences through the critical race theory lens. *Hamline Journal of Public Law & Policy, 27*, 55–76.

Samhan, H. H. (1999). Not quite White: Race classification and the Arab-American experience. In M. Suleiman (Ed.), *Arabs in America: Building a new future* (pp. 209–226). Philadelphia, PA: Temple University Press.

Shaheen, J. G. (1985). Media coverage of the Middle East: Perception and foreign policy. *The Annals of the American Academy of Political and Social Science, 482*(1), 160–175. https://doi.org/10.1177/0002716285482001010.

Shaheen, J. G. (2001). *Reel bad Arabs: How Hollywood vilifies a people*. New York: Olive Branch Press.

Shakir, E. (1997). *Bint Arab: Arab and Arab-American women in the United States*. Westport, CT: Greenwood Publishing Group.

Suleiman, M. F. (2000). *Teaching about Arab Americans: What social studies teachers should know*. Retrieved from http://eric.ed.gov/?id=ED442714

Wingfield, M. (2006). Arab Americans: Into the multicultural mainstream. *Equity & Excellence in Education, 39*, 253–266. https://doi.org/10.1080/10665680600788453.

Wingfield, M., & Karaman, B. (2009). *Arab stereotypes and American educators*. Retrieved June 10, 2019, from https://www.adc.org/arab-stereotypes-and-american-educators/

Wingfield, M., & Salam, S. (1993). *Working with school systems: Educational outreach and action guide* (p. 24). Washington, DC: American Arab Anti-Discrimination Committee.

Arab American Youth and Discrimination Post-9/11

Introduction

Since their immigration to the United States, Arabs in America have experienced stereotyping and discrimination, especially through the mainstream media and American governmental policies. The terrorist attacks of 9/11 were not the beginning of stereotyping and discrimination against Arab Americans. Researchers propose that 9/11 was a rather a turning point for the Arab experience in America. Specifically, the events turned Arab Americans from invisible to "glaringly conspicuous" (Salaita, 2005, p. 149). The attacks did not alter the American attitudes toward Arabs but instead reinforced attitudes that had existed for decades prior to 9/11 (Salaita, 2005). This chapter provides historical background of discrimination in the United States, beginning with the 9/11 attacks, to inform the school context for Arab American youth. The dialogue illustrates how preexisting stereotypes and misconceptions were magnified following the terrorist attacks. Research describing the specific accounts of Arab Americans in various communities are presented. This chapter provides context of how discrimination against Arab Americans has infiltrated various societal factors, including both local and federal government policies, the workforce, housing and lending opportunities, education systems, and in the general public domain. This greater context is presented to provide the background knowledge for how the K-12 school system arrived to its current status in terms of Arab cultures and youth. It is critical to understand the various discrimination experiences that Arab American youth encounter in their greater environments in order to truly understand their school experiences.

R. Tabbah, *Arab American Youth*, Advancing Responsible Adolescent Development, https://doi.org/10.1007/978-3-030-66804-4_4

Discrimination in the Post-9/11 Era

Arab American cultures have been historically misunderstood and misrepresented through media and various other sources (Abu El-Haj, 2006; Al-Hazza & Lucking, 2005; Awad & Amayreh, 2016; Harb, 2016; Wingfield, 2006); however, since the 9/11 terrorist attacks, negative images and stereotypes of Arabs and their cultures have increasingly permeated the media and the American society as a whole (Harb, 2016; Seikaly, 2001). For example, Shaheen (2003) examined the various stereotypes of Arabs exhibited in over 900 films. The most common portrayals of Arab men were found to be "brute murderers, sleazy rapists, religious fanatics, oil-rich dimwits, and abusers of women" (Shaheen, 2003, p. 172).

One of the most common misconceptions is the interchangeability of the terms "Arab" and "Muslim" (Al-Hazza & Lucking, 2005). Arab American is a category overarching individuals with diverse religious practices and various demographic factors, such as racial, national, dialectal, and political backgrounds (Hakim-Larson & Menna, 2016). Therefore, this particular misconception disregards the heterogeneity of this ethnic group (Suleiman, 2000). After 9/11, the misconception that all Arabs are Muslims—and vice versa—was further perpetuated, due to the majority of the terrorists being Arabs of Muslim faith. This incident also further intertwined the constructs of "Arab" and "Muslim" (Amer & Kayyali, 2016). Abu El-Haj (2006) provided a powerful description of the phenomenon of the Arab experience:

> In the discursive realms of politics, popular media, and academia, the notion of *culture* continually recasts Arabs and other Muslims outside of the confines of civilization, enemies of freedom, tolerance, and pluralism. Of significance for this historical moment is the extra burden that Islam bears within this discourse of culture, a burden imposed in both popular and academic venues. For it is Islam that is posited as most culturally "Other," inimical to Western values and traditions in an essential clash of civilizations. (p. 19)

Arab culture has generally been portrayed in a negative light throughout history; however, after 9/11, portrayals only seemed to worsen. Arabs and Arab Americans were labeled and portrayed further in the media as terrorists, the common enemy, and "other" (Abu El-Haj, 2006; Wingfield, 2006). Abu El-Haj (2006) discussed the cultural complexities of Arab Americans and argued that the mainstream media uses Arab culture to explain behaviors and norms of the Arab American people: "Arab culture is represented as a static set of traditions, values, norms, and practices to which Arabs adhere. Culture becomes the explanation for all kinds of behaviors from the exotic to the inexplicable. Culture explains everything from Arabs' legendary hospitality to their alleged hostility to democracy" (p. 20). Abu El-Haj continued with an example of how culture was used to explain the reactions of Arabs to the incidents of Abu Ghraib detainees in Iraq. The media claimed that men were humiliated by the interrogation practices because of their cultural beliefs against nudity, sexuality, and homosexuality. These commentators acted as if they would have been less humiliated had these practices been inflicted on the US citizens (Abu El-Haj, 2006).

Baker and Shryock (2009) stated that Arabs are often politically associated with radical, anti-American politics. In reality, most are socially conservative, hold highly positive views of American society, and have the ambition to participate in mainstream politics. According to Baker and Shryock (2009), the war on terror that followed the attacks raised questions regarding the values, sympathies, and loyalties of Arab and Muslim Americans, which subjected them to intense public scrutiny, backlash, and government surveillance. Research showed that following 9/11, only 46% of all Americans viewed Arab Americans positively (Traugott, Groves, & Kennedy, 2002), and whites and blacks in the Detroit region preferred to keep more of a social distance from Arab Americans than any other group (Farley, Krysan, & Couper, 2006).

Arab Americans have been victims of racial profiling before 9/11. However, since the attacks, racial profiling has increased tremendously. Saloom (2005) reported that 80% of Americans were opposed to racial profiling before the attacks. After the attacks, 60% of the American population supported racial profiling, especially in the case of Arab Americans. Advocators believed that profiling was necessary to prevent another attack and that doing so might have prevented 9/11 in the first place. If a person "looked" like an Arab (or a Muslim), then it would be necessary to profile them. Consequently, people who were neither Arab nor Muslim but had proximity to what is perceived to be an Arab or Muslim identity were profiled (Saloom, 2005). For example, Indian Sikhs who wore turbans were profiled because the turban is commonly associated with Arabs.

Immediately following 9/11, the US government established and implemented policies, such as the Patriot Acts, which allowed the surveillance of all Americans in the name of national security yet singled out Arabs and Muslims. This created a sense of fear and anxiety among visitors and immigrants from majority Muslim countries (Jamal, 2008). Jamal (2008) discussed the anti-Muslim backlash that followed this government scrutiny after 9/11. For example, passengers refused to board airplanes with individuals who appeared to be Muslim (Jamal, 2008). In addition, 2 years following the attacks, from 2001 to 2003, the Council on American Islamic Relations reported a 300% increase in hate crimes against Muslim Americans (Jamal, 2008). Furthermore, between 2004 and 2005, there was an additional 50% increase in hate crimes reported (Jamal, 2008). Jamal (2008) also reported on results from the Detroit Arab American Study (DAAS) conducted in 2003 regarding the willingness of individuals to support increased surveillance of the US citizens to ensure national security. The DAAS compared the results between Arab Americans and the general population.

When asked about trading some civil liberties to curb terrorism (47% of Arab Americans; 55% of general population) and supporting increased surveillance of the US citizens (56% of Arab Americans; 52% of general population), both the groups responded with similar support (Jamal, 2008). Forty-nine percent of the general population supported increasing surveillance of Arab Americans specifically, while only 17% of Arab Americans supported this.

When asked about upholding the detention of suspicious Arabs and Muslims even without sufficient evidence, 41% of the general population were in favor, while only 12% of Arab Americans were in favor (Jamal, 2008). Twenty-three percent of the general population was in support of increased police powers to stop and search Arabs and Muslims compared to 8% of Arab Americans supporting this action. Jamal (2008) speculated that the reasoning behind such popular support from the general population stems from the racialization or "otherization" of Arabs and Muslims in the mainstream American culture: "This racialization process essentially sees Muslims and Arabs as different from and inferior to whites, potentially violent and threatening, and therefore deserving of policies that target them as a distinct group of people and criminalize them without evidence of criminal activity" (p. 116). This process facilitates an ideology of "us" against "them" (Jamal, 2008). Furthermore, Americans who support infringing the rights and civil liberties of Arab Americans do so because of the various misperceptions and stereotypes they hold about this entire group (Jamal, 2008).

Various researchers have studied the Arab American experience post-9/11. Cainkar (2008) conducted a study with a sample of 102 Arab Muslims in Chicago. Forty-five percent were female. The majority of the sample was middle class (62%) while 18% were low income and 20% upper middle class and wealthy. Ages ranged from 19 to over 50 years. Education levels included high school or less (14%), some college or BS/BA (43%), and postgraduate (42%). Twenty-nine percent were born in the United States. The participants were asked if they had experienced discrimination since the 9/11 terrorist attacks. Fifty-three percent responded yes, while the remainder responded that they had not. Of the 53% reporting discrimination, 39% reported experiencing discrimination in places of employment, 22% in public spaces, 11% in schools, 11% with law enforcement, 9% with commercial transactions, 9% in government offices, 7% in airports/airplanes, and 6% in civil society institutions. The author reported that these responses were based strictly on the definition of discrimination as "being denied something or treated in a different way than others." Many of the respondents did not interpret hate speech, feeling unsafe, fearing removal from the United States, or having to change one's name to avoid prejudice as discrimination (Cainkar, 2008). One Palestinian-born male taxi driver stated,

> I can feel too much discrimination in people's eyes when they gaze or stare at me after realizing I'm Arabian. Actually my appearance is kind of tricky. I'm very white, so at the first glance people would think I'm American or belong to some other nationality, therefore, they treat me nicely. But, when I tell them I'm Arabian, their looks would change suddenly…In the past, I gave my business card to customers to call me whenever they need a ride, but they never did. It is only after I changed my Arabian name to be American that I have started to receive many calls from my customers. (p. 71)

Cainkar (2008) reported that the majority of respondents reported verbal harassment after 9/11 taking different forms, depending on the context of the situation. These behaviors largely occurred in public spaces where Arabs were seen as foreigners. They included being spat or sneezed upon and threatened with harm. One Chicago-born female expressed:

> We were driving and some teenagers shouted to us, "go back to your country. We need to get rid of you guys, kill you off. (p.72)

The second avenue for harassment was public schools (Cainkar, 2008), including the K-12 system and higher education institutions. Cainkar (2008) stated that schools have been a site for discrimination long before 9/11 and that pedagogical bias against Arabs and Muslims is taught through the school system. One study participant in community college reported:

> On 9/11 I was the only Arab in the class. We were watching TV and the teacher's way of dealing with me changed. He showed pictures of Osama bin Laden and said [pointing to the respondent], "Ask him if you have any questions." (p. 72)

Cainkar (2008) further discussed how the results showed that discrimination against Arabs and Muslims in school settings has been essentially institutionalized and that this is especially true where Arabs and Muslims are a significant minority population. One female teacher participant stated:

> The day after 9/11 I was in the lunchroom and one of my colleagues said he saw a woman at the grocery store "with that thing on her head" and he wanted to hit her. Another colleague said "that would be stupid, they did not do it," and another colleague said, "how do you know that, those people who did it were living here." I got up and left. I did not say anything. I was angry, and at the same time angry at myself for not having guts. After that, I was confiding in one of my friends what I felt and she said "if someone like you was next to me on an airplane, I'd get nervous. (p. 73)

The participants also reported experiencing discrimination in commercial transaction settings, particularly in primarily white suburban areas (Cainkar, 2008). An example presented by a Kuwaiti-born female stated:

> I was at Linens and Things in Naperville with my friend and my curtain rod was hanging over the cart. I turned to the guy behind me to apologize for my rod (it did not touch him). I apologized and he said "turn around and don't talk to me." I said "someone woke up on the wrong side of the bed." He said "It's none of your business what side of the bed I woke up on. Why don't you wake up and go back where you came from." I was just floored. (p. 74)

Some of the participants reported attacks on their homes as well (Cainkar, 2008). A Palestinian-born male respondent reported:

> Well, my van in front of my house was covered with eggs several times, about one or two months ago. I didn't report it…also some garbage was put in our mailbox, like ice cream cones and wrappers, stuff like that…Once we called the police because it wasn't just the cars but also the house! They pelted the door with eggs, so I called the Oak Lawn police and he came and looked around. I showed him above the door and the van, and I wasn't happy with it and he said "Well, maybe these are kids" and I said, "Yeah, I know they aren't adults but they did it on purpose, not just because they were just having fun because it's only my house and my car." On the street, there are so many cars parked but only my cars were the ones hit. He said, "I recommend that you have a garage," and I said, "Yes, I do." He said I should put the cars in the garage and I asked him "Officer, what should I do with my door? Put it in the garage too?" (p. 74)

The study participants also reported discrimination in the work setting and job application process with the latter discrimination being triggered by either names or looks (Cainkar, 2008). A Libyan-born female who migrated to the United States before the age of 10 years described her experience:

> Besides the physical and verbal abuse, I applied for a job and I feel that it's not just that I'm imagining it. They said, "We don't know if we want someone who covers." Obviously, this is illegal but this was when I was going to school and I was trying to get a job in retail. For example, "It's not part of the image we want to have, especially now being a negative connotation and with you covering and the whole post-9/11 thing." In that regard, I have absolutely been discriminated against pre-9/11 but especially post-9/11. I went to talk to the corporate manager of that retail chain and said it was uncalled for. They basically apologized and offered me a job but I didn't want to work there with other people who probably felt the same way. Someone who's not working in the shop but at the headquarters is different. Originally, I did talk to a lawyer and they were going to go into it but I didn't go further than that. (p. 75)

Cainkar (2008) indicated that the majority of participants reported not feeling safe in certain places in the American society. This feeling of lack of safety was also gendered because women, especially those who wear hijab, or headscarves, that reported this feeling more than men (Cainkar, 2008). These places for women were largely connected to whiteness, or areas that were predominantly white. Women reported suburban shopping centers and malls as being frequent venues of stares and insults. The majority of participants reported that they no longer feel secure in the United States, and they fear a mass deportation, revocation of citizenship, or internment camps.

Naber (2008) conducted an ethnographic research study among Arab immigrants and Arab Americans in the San Francisco Bay Area between September 2002 and September 2003. This research took place among two Arab/Arab American community networks. The first included recent Arab Muslim immigrants and refugees from Iraq, Yemen, Palestine, and North Africa living in poverty. The second community included middle- and upper-class professionals who were majority first and second generation and consisted of both Muslims and Christians from the Levant region. Naber (2008) reported that the research consisted of interviews and observations of study participants, which included 30 board members representing eight religious, civil rights, and community-based organizations that serve Arabs/Arab Americans among their constituencies. The author interviewed and observed 50 community members from various class, generational, religious backgrounds, and countries of origin in the Arab world. Naber (2008) also conducted interviews with six lawyers who focused on community-based efforts in response to anti-Arab/South Asian/Muslim backlash in the San Francisco Bay Area after 9/11.

The interviews revealed that the "terrorist profile" set forth by the Bush administration was arbitrary and had the potential to single-out a wide range of individuals, including Arab and Pakistani Muslims, non-Arab/non-South Asian Muslims; Christians and Jews; aliens, permanent residents, and citizens; and young men in addition to teenagers and the elderly (Naber, 2008). For example, one immigrant rights lawyer stated:

> It was mostly Muslims [who] were detained, but there were Christians among them. There was an Iranian Armenian family. There were Jews among them. The gamut. The ones that look darker were more targeted. There was a particular age group I saw- twenty-somethings and forty-somethings, but I also saw sixteen-year-olds and I saw sixty-four-year-olds" (p. 287).

Interviews with community members revealed that post-9/11 hate crimes and harassment in the public domain largely targeted individuals who resembled those of the "Arab/Middle Eastern/Muslim" identity constructed by the government and media, including types of names, appearances, and countries of origin (Naber, 2008). Naber (2008) found that these identity markers were related to the various hate crimes and forms of violence that were reported by participants in the public domain, including schools, on the bus, at work, at home, and on the streets. The first theme the author identified within participants' narratives was that particular names, such as Mohammed and Osama, instigated harassment. One Muslim American youth group leader reported an incident where school kids would frequently shout, "Look, Mohammed the terrorist is coming!" when a young man named Mohammed would join the playground (p. 290). Another father expressed the difficulties he and his wife had when naming their son:

> After September 11 no one would have thought about naming their son Mohammed in this country if they wanted him to be treated like a normal person. We thought about what would happen to our son in school, and how he would be discriminated against growing up. But we felt that this is our religion and our culture, and long before September 11 we decided that if we had a second son, we would name him Mohammed. We decided not to change what we stood for, but imagine what happens when your neighbor says, "what is that cute little boy's name?" You say "Mohammed" and they say, "Oh…" This is how September 11 impacted even the relationship between you and your neighbor. (p. 291)

Even Christian Arabs/Arab Americans were similarly targeted because of their names being associated with the notion of "enemy of the nation" (p. 291). This was particularly the case when they held Arabic names, which, Naber (2008) stated, speaks to the conflation of "Arab" and "Muslim" constructs. Several of these participants changed their names to English names. For example, one youth group leader at a Roman Catholic Arab American church reported that they changed their son's name from Osama to Sam after he was repeatedly called "Muslim terrorist" (p. 291). Naber (2008) also discussed how some of the narratives revealed an association between particular names with Muslim masculinity and terrorism. Moreover, this masculinity was associated with inherent violence toward women. As a cab driver described a passenger's reaction to his name, Mohammed:

> Once, a woman got in my car. She looked at me, then read my name, then asked me if I was Muslim. When I said "yes" she replied, "how many girls have you killed today?" (p. 293)

The next theme found within stories of harassment was among women who wore a hijab, or headscarf. Naber (2008) found that, while federal government policies largely targeted men, women were more likely targeted through hate crimes and harassment in the public. The author provides an example from a Muslim American woman community activist:

> Women who wear *hijab* were more of a target because they're more visible than Muslim men in public. The awareness that they were in more danger and were more impacted than men could be seen by all of the events that were organized in solidarity with veiled women in response to the backlash. There were days of solidarity organized across the nation. (p. 293)

Results showed that several women were fired from their jobs for wearing headscarves. Community activists working with Arab Muslim youth reported several cases of girls who wore the headscarf receiving harassment on the bus, at school, and in the street, which included people trying to pull of their headscarves. In addition, there were several cases where women contemplated taking off their headscarves. A university student reported:

> I knew I had to prepare for at least some kind of backlash because I was visually identifiable. My mother, who doesn't cover, specifically told me "Don't go outside for a month or two. Wait till things die down." I was like, "I shouldn't hide. I shouldn't be scared or restrain my lifestyle because of ignorance." (p. 294)

The third theme found was the instigation of harassment and association of terrorism by men with beards, dark skin, and, in some cases, wore a particular form of religious dress. Results demonstrated that male participants in the study with this appearance were the most severely concerned for their safety (Naber, 2008). Results also showed that non-Muslim South Asian men—such as Sikhs—were often misidentified as Muslims and targeted in harassment and hate crimes.

The final theme found by Naber (2008) was the association of specific countries of origin and potential terrorism. The author found that these countries of origin tended to be the ones that the Bush administration often referred to as "terrorist-harboring or training countries." Moreover, experience with harassment was aggravated when the individual simultaneously showed some sense of solidarity with any of these countries. In these cases, participants experienced harassment and violence in attempt to silence their political dissent. An example was presented of a Palestinian woman who wore a kufiyah, or a scarf representing Palestinian resistance, on a daily basis and posted a sticker of a Palestinian flag on a window near the front door of her house:

> I walked out [our door] and saw all this graffiti. I didn't know...Should I be afraid? Angry? Then I looked at the sidewalk and saw "Kill Arabs" in big blocks right in front of our house. The graffiti was all done in black spray paint. On top of the door, it said "Die pig" in big block letters over where the Palestinian flag is. On the side wall were the words, "Die pig." (p. 299)

Naber (2008) continued describing that the perpetrator returned to this participant's home five times. During one incident, the perpetrator threw feces and garbage all over her front door. Another subject described her experience on a university campus:

> We were having a memorial for victims of the Israeli massacre of the refugee camp Jenin. Two people came over to disrupt the event. They were saying, "Go blow yourself up" to a group of Arab American students who were there. (p. 300)

The Detroit Arab American Study Team (DAAST) developed a survey study to examine the experiences of adults of Arab or Chaldean descent in the post-9/11 era (DAAST, 2009). The survey study consisted of two separate samples described by Baker and Shryock (2009). The Detroit Arab American Study (DAAS) surveyed a sample of 1016 Arab Americans from the Michigan counties of Wayne, Oakland, and Macomb regarding their experiences post-9/11, while the Detroit Area Study

(DAS) surveyed a sample of 508 adult subjects from the general population in the same three counties. The total sample included 1524 surveys. Both studies were designed so that samples were representative of the population in these three counties. The Arab American sample from the DAAS was compared to the general population sample from the DAS.

To participate in the DAS survey, individuals were required to be 18 years or older and reside in any of the three counties cited above. To be eligible for the DAAS, participants had to be 18 years of age or older, live in households in the three-county Detroit region during the survey period of July to December 2003, and identify themselves as Arab or Chaldean. Baker and Shryock (2009) reported that identification of Arabs was rather difficult, since the idea about who is Arab and how the identity should be defined are controversial. For example, while language is frequently mentioned, many Arab Americans do not speak Arabic well or at all, and some people who reject the Arab identity only speak Arabic (Baker & Shryock, 2009). Furthermore, an individual might not identify themselves as Arab and would rather be called American, and still will watch Arabic satellite television and attend a church where most speak Arabic (Baker & Shryock, 2009). Others use a specific national label, such as Lebanese or Palestinian (Baker & Shryock, 2009). Many do not identify themselves consistently as Arab even though they come from Arab countries, speak Arabic, and share cultural traits with Arabs (Baker & Shryock, 2009). Due to the variety of identification factors, the researchers decided to incorporate a more flexible and inclusive approach to determine eligibility, which consisted of asking potential participants if there was anyone in the household who had parents, grandparents, or ancestors who were Arab or Chaldean.

Howell and Jamal (2009) examined the post-9/11 data on backlash from the DAAS. According to the DAAS results, 15% of respondents disclosed that they personally had a bad experience due to their race or ethnicity after 9/11. Sixty-one percent of these discriminatory acts included verbal insults and threats. Forty-three percent of respondents reported worrying about the future facing their families in the United States following the attacks. Respondents born in the United States (19%) reported more bad experiences than did foreign-born (14%) respondents; however, foreign-born respondents reported significantly more worry about their future than were United States born. Muslim respondents reported significantly higher incidents of bad experiences and worry about the future than did their Christian counterparts. Howell and Jamal (2009) reported that a common theme among the interviews was a concern for the degradation of civil liberties and the profiling of Arab communities by law enforcement and the media.

The Arab American Institute Foundation (AAIF, 2002) conducted a survey study regarding Arab Americans behaviors and attitudes post-9/11. Results from this study were also compared to the AAIF's survey study conducted in 2001 immediately after the 9/11 terror attacks. Phone interviews were conducted with 505 participants chosen at random nationwide who identified as having Middle Eastern or Arabic-speaking backgrounds. Three-fourths of the sample was born in the United States and 89% held United States citizenship. Eighty-one participants spoke English at home. Religious affiliation of the sample included: 63% Christians, 24%

Muslims, and 13% other or no religious affiliation. Demographics for this sample in terms of occupation were reportedly found to represent the United States Census data on this characteristic with 36% reporting some form of professional or managerial job. In addition, results from the survey showed that 10% were teachers, 7% were homemakers, 22% reported membership in unions, and 34% owned or operated a business. Household income above $50,000 was reported by two out of three respondents, while 16% reported incomes below $25,000. In order to gauge identification, participants were asked, "How are you most likely to describe yourself?" Thirty-nine percent identified as Arab American while 21% identified by their country of origin, 12% as both Arab American and country of origin, and one in four used neither to identify themselves. Demographic results also showed that United States-born respondents were less likely (36%) to identify themselves as Arab American than those born elsewhere (49%). Half of the American citizens who were not born in the United States (51%) describe themselves as Arab American, while 44% of permanent residents identified themselves by country of origin.

The following questions were asked to each participant regarding discrimination before and after 9/11 (AAIF, 2002): (1) Have you personally experienced discrimination in the past because of your ethnicity? (2) Since the terrorist attacks on the United States on September 11, have you personally experienced discrimination because of your ethnicity? (3) Do you know anyone of Arabic ethnicity or with an Arabic-speaking background who has experienced discrimination since the terrorist attacks on September 11? (4) Have any of your children or any member of your household experienced discrimination since the terrorist attacks on September 11?

In order to measure where discrimination was experienced, participants answered the following questions (AAIF, 2002): (1) Have you experienced such discrimination (in the past) in any of the following? (at school; at work; from friends, acquaintances, neighbors; other; not sure) (2) Have you experienced such discrimination (since the terrorist attacks on the United States on September 11) in any of the following? (at school; at work; from friends, acquaintances, neighbors; other; not sure).

Results from the 2002 survey study (AAIF, 2002) revealed that 20% personally experienced discrimination because of their ethnicity since 9/11. Twenty percent also reported that their children or a member in their household has experienced discrimination. Forty percent reported that they know someone of Arab ethnicity or an Arabic-speaking background who has experienced an increase in discrimination following the attacks. The AAIF (2002) reported that US-born Arabs and those born outside of the United States equally experienced discrimination in the past prior to 9/11 with an equal 30% each. Results from this post-9/11 survey showed that Arab Americans born outside of the United States reported experiencing more personal discrimination at 27% than did their US-born counterparts at 17%. Fifty-four percent of 18- to 29-year olds reported experiencing discrimination, while the majority of those above the age of 30 years were more likely to report no experiences with personal discrimination. When comparing religious characteristics to experiences of discrimination, Arab American Protestants and Muslims were on average (43%) more likely than Eastern Orthodox or Catholics (24%) to have experienced personal discrimination in the past. After the attacks, Arab American Muslims at 46% were much more likely to report personal experiences with discrimination than Arab Americans of any other religious affiliation, including 14% of Protestants and 10% of Catholics.

Regarding where discrimination was experienced, in the past, Arab Americans reported that discrimination occurred at work (29%), at school (30%), among friends, neighbors, and acquaintances (25%). After 9/11, however, respondents reported that discrimination is less prevalent at school (21%), while remaining the same at work and among friends, neighbors, and acquaintances. They reported a sense that discrimination is more likely to occur in other public spaces such as airports and shopping malls. The majority of those who reported an increase in discrimination at school were participants aged 18–24 years (36%). On average at 37%, respondents who were business owners and those not born in the United States reported being discriminated against at work.

When asked about their perceptions regarding the profiling of Arab Americans since 9/11, more than 75% of respondents perceived that there has been an increase in profiling, which was a 9% increase from 2001 (AAIF, 2002). Twelve percent reported perceptions of profiling being the same, 3% felt there was less profiling, and 7% were not sure. Among the sample that was most likely to report an increase were 90% of 18- to 29-year olds and more than 80% of US-born respondents.

Participants were then asked: "How worried are you about the long-term effects of discrimination against Arab Americans: very worried, somewhat worried, or not worried?" (AAIF, 2002). Sixty-three percent reported being very or somewhat worried about the long-term effects, while 37% were not worried. Among the respondents reporting that they were very or somewhat worried were four in five Muslims and an average of 73% of 18- to 49-year olds and Arab Americans born outside of the United States. Participants were also asked if they were reassured by President Bush's comments and conduct toward Arab Americans following 9/11. Fifty-four percent reported feeling reassured, while 35% were not reassured. The AAIF (2002) reported that this was a significant decrease from 2001 perceptions where 90% of Arab Americans were reassured by the president's response. Among the group that was not reassured in 2002, most likely to feel this way were an average of 45% of 18–34 years of age and 58% of Muslims.

The American Arab Anti-Discrimination Committee (ADC) Research Institute conducted a survey study on the experiences of Arab Americans in the year following the 9/11 terrorist attacks (Ibish, 2003). The time period covered by this report included September 11, 2001 through October 11, 2002. Airline discrimination and airport profiling significantly increased during this time period with over 80 cases documented. One case example presented occurred on December 18, 2001, in the Baltimore Washington International Airport in Maryland:

> A 17-year-old Muslim-American high school student from Virginia was passing through security when suddenly an airport security guard stopped her. "Hey, you need to take that off," the guard called out, referring to her hijab. "Why do I have to take off my head cover?" the girl asked, when suddenly nearby military personnel approached her. The sight of the guards in camouflage, carrying combat rifles intimidated the frightened teenager and she quickly took off her hijab. A Muslim airport employee rushed to her assistance upon

> witnessing the scene. The employee informed the guard that it was wrong to force the student to remove her headscarf in public. (p. 30)

Ibish (2003) reported that a new set of government policies were established following 9/11 that reintroduced ethnic and national origin discrimination for the first time in decades. According to Ibish (2003), these policies discriminated against Arabs and Muslims through alien registration, visa screening procedures, tracking foreign nationals already in the country, selectively deporting Middle Eastern so-called absconders, and secretly detaining and deporting individuals for minor visa violations, often times without due process (p. 31). Additionally, the survey revealed an insurmountable number of reports of hate crimes and discrimination throughout 41 states and the District of Columbia directed at Arab Americans and those perceived to be Arab American (Ibish, 2003). The ADC confirmed over 700 incidents of violence in the first 9 weeks following 9/11. Furthermore, in the first 9 months of 2002, 165 reports were documented and 66% of these involved physical and psychological attacks. Twenty-seven percent of claims involved acts of vandalism and arson, 22% involved hate mail, threats and bomb threats, 16% involved beatings and physical attacks, and 1% murders (Ibish, 2003). Physical attacks reportedly involved battery or destruction of property and occurred mostly during the week of September 11 and 18, 2001 with 54% of battery reports, 67% of vandalism, and five of the suspected or confirmed hate crime murders (Ibish, 2003). A case summary of vandalism occurred in the Fall of 2001 in Chelmsley Wood, Alabama:

> A Muslim mother and her two children, ages 17 and 12, were repeatedly harassed and their property damaged by a mob of vandals. Since the September 11 attacks, the family has seen their car fire bombed, their front door kicked in and the tires on another car slashed. They often hear slurs and vulgarity directed at them yelled from outside their home. Officers set up a camera in the family's home to try to protect them, but that did not stop the attacks on their car. (p. 49)

An example of battery reported during this time period involved an incident on September 11, 2001 in Ardsley, New York:

> An Arab-American deli owner was asked if he was Arab by one customer. When he responded affirmatively, the customer cursed and yelled at him. The customer then sprayed the deli owner with pepper spray when he attempted to escort him out of the store. (p. 60)

Ibish (2003) reported an influx of employment discrimination from September 2001 to October 2002, which was four times the rate of previous years. These incidents occurred across the United States with the greatest numbers coming, respectively, from California, Virginia, Michigan, and New York (Ibish, 2003). Employment discrimination experiences were reportedly based on national origin, religion, citizenship status, race, and political opinion. Examples of employment discrimination follow. In September 2001 in Fontana, California:

> A Muslim high school senior working at a fast-food restaurant was the repeated target of bias jokes from both his coworkers and his manager. At first, coworkers taunted him, asking him why his "cousins" destroyed the World Trade Center. Sometime later, his manager began teasing him as well. "Hey, we're going to have to check you for bombs," the manager joked, often in front of other employees. Days later, he was fired after he accidentally threw

away a paper cup that the manager was using. Management said he was let go for "performance deficiencies." (pp. 92–93)

Ibish (2008), through the American Arab Anti-Discrimination Committee (ADC) Research Institute, compiled a subsequent report regarding the various hate crimes and discrimination against Arab Americans from 2003 through 2007. Results indicated that, while there was a decrease of incidents during this time compared to immediately following 9/11, occurrences were still significantly more frequent than pre-9/11. The ADC documented more than 700 violent incidents directed toward Arab Americans in the first few weeks following 9/11. Violent hate crimes were defined as "acts of violence or specific and credible threats of violence" (p. 11). During the 2003–2007 time period, there were between 120 and 130 hate crimes documented per year. This is compared to between 80 and 90 per year in the late 1990s. One case study discussed occurred in New Jersey in 2005 and involved the forceful eviction and beating of an Arab American male:

> An Arab-American man in New Jersey had been renting a room although he had allegedly faced tensions with the landlord in the past. One rainy night, the man was locked out of his room and the landlord refused to let him in. He stayed out in the rain until 7 am when a hooded man walked up to him and began to kick and beat him. He was dragged to the porch and the attacker yelled a number of insults including, "you---Arab, what the---do you think you are? This is my house! No Arabs allowed here." On the porch, the landlord got involved as well, as it turned out the attacker was his son. He later pulled out a knife and threatened the Arab-American man, and said he would kill him if he did not move out of "his house" within an hour. While local police did not seem to react, the ADC Legal Department contacted the FBI that looked into the matter but did not opened an investigation. (p. 13)

Ibish (2008) reported about 80 incidents of airport discrimination and racial profiling at airports, as well as an increase in border detentions and delays following the 9/11 attacks. Such incidents were exacerbated by "watch lists" developed by the US government as part of national security and law enforcement efforts where Arab Americans encountered "false positives" associated with these lists (Ibish, 2008). These problems reportedly mostly involved officers with the Customs and Border Protection services and highly occurred on the border of the United States and Canada, especially crossing through the border near Detroit, Michigan. For example, in September 2006 in New York:

> Employees of U.S. Customs and Border Protection at New York's JFK International Airport mistreated a mother and her children, returning from a family vacation in Jordan. They were made to wait two and a half hours until called for questioning. The incident allegedly came from a decision by CBP authorities at JFK to hold and question all or most passengers on flights arriving from Arab countries, including U.S. citizens. (p. 20)

In June 2002, the Department of Justice established and enforced the National Security Entry-Exit Registration System (NSEERS) which required male visitors, 16 years and older, from specified countries, along with other secret criteria, to be fingerprinted, photographed, and questioned by immigration officers (Ibish, 2008). The "domestic call-in" phase of the NSEERS required men from 25 different Arab and Muslim countries to report to immigration offices around the country for fingerprinting, photographs, and questioning. Ibish (2008) reported that about 14,000 men who actually complied with these procedures were placed in removal proceedings. Parts of the NSEERS were discontinued in December 2003; however, the program was modified in December 2004, and the remaining features included departure registration, registration at ports of entry, and the potential for the re-initiation of domestic call-ins and enforcement action based on the information collected through the program (Ibish, 2008).

Throughout the period of 2003 and 2007, Ibish (2008) reported that Arabs/Arab Americans faced a significant amount of discrimination and abuse in jails, prisons, and immigration detention centers. Discrimination in these scenarios involved denial of religious accommodations and religious discrimination, transfers with either no notice or insufficient notice, and incidents where Arab/Arab American children were "unjustly, unnecessarily, and indefensibly" detained in immigration detention facilities (p. 28). Experiences with state and local police misconduct involved racial, ethnic, or religious slurs and unjustified arbitrary use of authority (Ibish, 2008). A case example presented occurred in May 2002 in North Providence, Rhode Island:

> An Arab-American mother and her daughter were approached by two North Providence police officers while they were ordering beverages at a drive through. With their guns drawn, the officers ordered them to get out of the car, only to change their minds and order them stay in the car with their hands on the dashboard. They allegedly used profane and ethnic language and spat while questioning them. After the officers let them go, the girl at the drive-through window and an older lady who worked there apologized and gave them their beverages. The officers never apologized for their behavior or the fear that they instilled. (p. 29)

One of the most significant forms of discrimination found within this time period was employment discrimination with about ten reports occurring per week (Ibish, 2008). Reports largely involved hostile work environments resulting from repeated slurs and abusive comments by coworkers and managers who focused on ethnic, racial, or religious identities (Ibish, 2008). Incidents occurred in both private and public sector employment environments.

More recent events involving the Arab Spring and the rise of ISIS in Iraq and Syria have further complicated socio-political issues in the media (Harb, 2016). The attacks in Paris, France in 2015 by ISIS (Almasy, Meilhan, & Bittermann, 2015) have left the American Arab Anti-Discrimination Committee (ADC) working diligently to dispel misconceptions being conveyed in the media (ADC, 2015). Furthermore, the Arab American Institute (AAI) conducted a recent poll revealing that views have only increased in negativity since their previous survey study in 2010, suggesting that there continue to be persistent and hostile portrayals of Arabs and Muslims in America (AAI, 2015).

Awad and Amayreh (2016) suggested that such negative stereotypes and portrayals likely lead to various forms of discrimination, including organizational and institutional. Experimental studies of evidence include Widner and Chicoine (2011) where the authors randomly assigned a typical white-sounding name or a typical Arab sounding name to two similar fictitious resumes. The authors sent these resumes to 265 jobs over a 15-month period. Results showed that an Arab male applicant needed to send two resumes for every one resume sent by a white applicant in order to receive a response for an interview through hiring staff (Widner & Chicoine, 2011). This finding was especially true for applications to an office managerial position compared to a customer service managerial position (Widner & Chicoine, 2011). This finding suggests that higher status positions corresponded to greater discrimination (Widner & Chicoine, 2011). Widner and Chicoine (2011) posited that discrimination against the perceived race/ethnicity of the applicant was the culprit of these results. In another study, Carpusor and Loges (2006) tested the effects of name-based ethnic stereotypes on housing discrimination. The authors sent 1115 inquiry email messages to apartment landlords in Los Angeles County over a 10-week period. They randomly assigned to each email one of three typically sounding names for Arab, African American, or white ethnicity. Results showed that for all rent categories, in both corporate and privately owned apartment complexes, African American and Arab names received significantly less positive responses than did the white name.

Awad and Amayreh (2016) also posited that negative stereotypes of Arabs have adverse consequences on intergroup relations and the way Arabs are treated. For example, Hitti (2013) conducted an experimental study among a sample of adolescents between the ages of 12 and 16 years. Results showed that those endorsing stereotypes against Arabs were less likely to be empathetic toward and socially inclusive of an Arab American character represented in a vignette. Studies have also shown that holding stereotypes and prejudice toward Arabs and Muslims may also cause anxiety and aggressive responses among those who carry these prejudices (Awad & Amayreh, 2016). A study by Lyons, Kenworthy, and Popan (2010) showed a significant correlation between increased anxiety and perceptions of Arabs as threatening in non-Arab participants.

Negative stereotypes and portrayals may be culturally conditioned in the minds and behaviors of the mainstream public toward Arabs. Cultural conditioning refers to the process by which people acquire attitudes and values that are passed on by society through avenues such as the media, government, and schools (Henderson, 1988). This process affects the way people think about and act toward others (Henderson, 1988). Henderson (1988) posited that this process is required to assimilate successfully into the community; nonetheless, cultural conditioning potentially hinders society by enabling individuals to follow their surroundings blindly. After the 9/11 terrorist attacks, this is increasingly true in the case of portrayal of Arabs in America. The majority of what the American public views in the media about Arabs and their culture is negative, and because they do not generally have contact with Arabs to contradict these images, the negative views usually prevail (Alsultany, 2008; Suleiman, 1996). In other words, the American people have been culturally conditioned to view Arab cultures and people in negative ways. Consequently, because Americans view Arabs negatively, it is difficult for Arabs in America to view themselves positively (Suleiman, 2000). This is especially true for adolescents as they begin to figure out who they are and where they belong.

Conclusion

This chapter provided an overview of the research regarding Arab American experiences with discrimination following the 9/11 terrorist attacks. The continued cultural conditioning of the mainstream public regarding stereotypes and misconceptions—which existed prior to 9/11—expanded after the attacks and manifested in their treatment of Arabs. The most common misconception is the interchangeability of the concepts "Arab" and "Muslim." This has led to the racialization of Islam, which essentially complicates matters for Arab Christians and of other practicing faiths. Discrimination against Arab Americans has found its way to multiple societal facets, including government policies, the workplace, housing and lending opportunities, education systems, and general public spaces. In summary, Arabs have been deprived of civil liberties and are racially profiled to the extent that non-Arabs who resemble what a stereotypical Arab looks like have been profiled. Negative images and stereotypes are rampant in Hollywood films, and these factors are exacerbated through politics and government policies. The prevalence of discrimination throughout general society calls for a thorough examination of the possible infiltration of such discrimination into the American education systems. Researchers suggest that such experiences potentially have a detrimental impact on developmental growth in Arab American youth (Al-Hazza & Bucher, 2010; Suleiman, 1996; Wingfield, 2006; Wingfield & Karaman, 2009).

References

AAI. (2015). *American attitudes toward Arabs and Muslims: 2015*. Retrieved September 15, 2019, from http://www.aaiusa.org/american_attitudes_toward_arabs_and_muslims_2015

AAIF. (2002). *Profiling and pride: Arab American attitudes and behavior since September 11*. Washington, DC: Arab American Institute Foundation.

Abu El-Haj, T. R. (2006). Race, politics, and Arab American youth: Shifting frameworks for conceptualizing educational equity. *Educational Policy, 20*, 13–34. https://doi.org/10.1177/0895904805285287.

ADC. (2015). *Refuting the myths in the Syrian and Iraqi refugee debate: ADC separates fact from fiction*. Retrieved September 20, 2019, from http://www.adc.org/2015/11/refuting-the-myths-in-the-syrian-and-iraqi-refugee-debate-adc-separates-fact-from-fiction/

Al-Hazza, T., & Bucher, K. T. (2010). Bridging a cultural divide with literature about Arabs and Arab Americans. *Middle School Journal, 41*, 4–11. https://doi.org/10.2307/23047567.

Al-Hazza, T., & Lucking, B. (2005). The minority of suspicion: Arab Americans. *MultiCultural Review, 14*, 32–38.

Almasy, S., Meilhan, P., & Bittermann, J. (2015). *Paris massacre: At least 128 killed in gunfire and blasts, French officials say*. Retrieved August 22, 2016, from http://www.cnn.com/2015/11/13/world/paris-shooting/

Alsultany, E. (2008). The prime-time plight of the Arab Muslim American after 9/11. In A. Jamal & N. Naber (Eds.), *Race and Arab Americans before and after 9/11* (pp. 204–228). Syracuse, NY: Syracuse University Press.

Amer, M. M., & Kayyali, R. A. (2016). Religion and religiosity: Christian and Muslim faiths, diverse practices, and psychological correlates. In M. M. Amer & G. H. Awad (Eds.), *Handbook of Arab American psychology*. New York: Routledge.

Awad, G. H., & Amayreh, W. M. (2016). Discrimination: Heightened prejudice post 9/11 and psychological outcomes. In M. M. Amer & G. H. Awad (Eds.), *Handbook of Arab American psychology* (pp. 63–75). New York: Routledge.

Baker, W., & Shryock, A. (2009). Citizenship and crisis. In DAAST (Ed.), *Citizenship and crisis: Arab Detroit after 9/11* (pp. 3–32). New York: Russell Sage Foundation.

Cainkar, L. (2008). Thinking outside the box: Arabs and race in the United States. In A. Jamal & N. Naber (Eds.), *Race and Arab Americans before and after 9/11: From invisible citizens to visible subjects* (pp. 46–80). Syracuse, NY: Syracuse University Press.

Carpusor, A. G., & Loges, W. E. (2006). Rental discrimination and ethnicity in names. *Journal of Applied Social Psychology, 36*(4), 934–952. https://doi.org/10.1111/j.0021-9029.2006.00050.x.

DAAST. (2009). Citizenship and crisis: Arab Detroit after 9/11. New York: Russel Sage Foundation.

Farley, R., Krysan, M., & Couper, M. (2006). *Attitudes about Arab Americans: Detroiters' views*. Paper presented at the Sixty-First Annual Conference of the American Association for Public Opinion Research, Montreal, Canada.

Hakim-Larson, J., & Menna, R. (2016). Acculturation and enculturation: Ethnic identity socialization process. In M. M. Amer & G. H. Awad (Eds.), *Handbook of Arab American psychology* (pp. 34–47). New York: Routledge.

Harb, C. (2016). The Arab region. In M. M. Amer & G. H. Awad (Eds.), *Handbook of Arab American psychology* (pp. 3–18). New York: Routledge.

Henderson, J. L. (1988). The cultural unconscious. *Quadrant, 21*(2), 7–16. Retrieved from https://quadrant.org.au/magazine/

Hitti, A. (2013). *Social exclusion in cultural context: Group norms, fairness, and stereotypes*. Doctoral dissertation, University of Maryland. Retrieved from http://hdl.handle.net/1903/14008

Howell, S., & Jamal, A. (2009). The aftermath of the 9/11 attacks. In DAAST (Ed.), *Citizenship and crisis: Arab Detroit after 9/11* (pp. 69–100). New York: Russell Sage Foundation.

Ibish, H. E. (2003). *Report on hate crimes and discrimination against Arab Americans: The post-September 11 Backlash September 11, 2001 - October 11, 2002*. Washington, DC: American Arab Anti-Discrimination Committee Research Institute.

Ibish, H. E. (2008). *Report on hate crimes and discrimination against Arab Americans 2003-2007*. Washington, DC: American Arab Anti-Discrimination Committee Research Institute.

Jamal, A. (2008). Civil liberties and the otherization of Arab and Muslim Americans. In A. Jamal & N. Naber (Eds.), *Race and Arab Americans before and after 9/11* (pp. 114–130). Syracuse, NY: Syracuse University Press.

Lyons, P. A., Kenworthy, J. B., & Popan, J. R. (2010). Ingroup identification and group-level narcissism as predictors of U.S. citizens' attitudes and behavior toward Arab immigrants. *Personality and Social Psychology Bulletin, 36*, 1267–1280. https://doi.org/10.1177/0146167210380604.

Naber, N. (2008). Look, Mohammed the terrorist is coming! In A. Jamal & N. Naber (Eds.), *Race and Arab Americans before and after 9/11* (pp. 276–304). Syracuse, NY: Syracuse University Press.

Salaita, S. (2005). Ethnic identity and imperative patriotism: Arab Americans before and after 9/11. *College Literature, 32*(2), 146–168.

Saloom, R. (2005). I know you are, but what am I? Arab-American experiences through the critical race theory lens. *Hamline Journal of Public Law & Policy, 27*, 55–76.

Seikaly, Z. A. (2001). At risk of prejudice: The Arab American community. *Social Education, 65*, 349–351. Retrieved from http://www.socialstudies.org/system/files/publications/se/6506/650604.html

Shaheen, J. G. (2003). Reel bad Arabs: How Hollywood vilifies a people. *The Annals of the American Academy of Political and Social Science, 588*, 171–193.

Suleiman, M. F. (1996). *Educating the Arab American child: Implications for teachers*. Retrieved from http://eric.ed.gov/?id=ED392864

Suleiman, M. F. (2000). *Teaching about Arab Americans: What social studies teachers should know*. Retrieved from http://eric.ed.gov/?id=ED442714

Traugott, M. W., Groves, R. M., & Kennedy, C. (2002). *How Americans responded: Public opinion after 9/11/01*. Paper presented at the Fifty-Seventh Annual AAPOR Conference, St. Pete Beach, FL.

Widner, D., & Chicoine, S. (2011). It' all in the name: Employment discrimination against Arab Americans. *Sociological Forum, 26*(4), 806–823.

Wingfield, M. (2006). Arab Americans: Into the multicultural mainstream. *Equity & Excellence in Education, 39*, 253–266. https://doi.org/10.1080/10665680600788453.

Wingfield, M., & Karaman, B. (2009). *Arab stereotypes and American educators*. Retrieved June 10, 2019, from https://www.adc.org/arab-stereotypes-and-american-educators/

Arab American Youth and Discrimination in the Education System

Introduction

The historical standard of misinformation and misrepresentation of Arab American cultures throughout mainstream society inevitably infiltrates the educational system environment. Schools tend to reproduce the structures that exist in the societies in which they operate. Essentially, schools do not exist in a vacuum. There is evidence that negative perceptions have led to various forms of discrimination regarding Arab American students in schools. Incidents did occur prior to 9/11 but rather infrequently; however, following the attacks, the number of incidents surged (Ibish, 2001). It is critical to understand the various discrimination experiences that Arab American adolescents encounter in their greater environments, especially in regard to the education system. Discrimination in schools may have dire consequences for adolescent development, similar to the effects of discrimination in mainstream public. This chapter discusses how discrimination in the mainstream context has generalized into the educational system in the United States for Arab youth. The text presents on the various forms of discrimination found in schools in general. The chapter then reverts to a discussion of specific studies documenting the discrimination experiences of Arab American youth in the school system.

Discrimination in the K-12 System

The Arab American student population is reportedly growing (Suleiman, 2001a); however, because Arab Americans are generally categorized under the Caucasian or white category, the group is underrepresented, and it is difficult to obtain an accurate count (Wingfield, 2006). Asi and Beaulieu (2013) estimate that 29% of Arab Americans are under the age of 18 years and 41% are under the age of 25 years, which constitutes a large population of school-aged Arab American youth. Although

R. Tabbah, *Arab American Youth*, Advancing Responsible Adolescent Development, https://doi.org/10.1007/978-3-030-66804-4_5

the Arab American student population is growing, they have not been largely represented in the literature relative to other ethnic minority groups (Nieto, 1996). Perhaps, this is because Arab Americans tend to achieve higher academically than most other ethnic groups (Banks, 2009). Although this population may succeed academically, these students face other challenges as a minority in the school system. Since the terrorist attacks of 9/11, there seems to be an increased need for research and culturally relevant information to help researchers and educators to better understand this ethnic group and to better serve youth and their families.

The literature refers to Arab American youth as "the invisible minority" (Al-Khatab, 1999; Nieto, 2000; Suleiman, 2001b). However, this population has been highly visible through negative images and stereotypes portrayed in the media (Nieto, 2000). These images are permeated in the minds of American society and have made their way into schools. The specific experiences in schools coming from the voices of Arab American youth have not been reported or researched extensively. Given the long history of discrimination with Arab Americans documented in the literature (Abu El-Haj, 2006; Awad & Amayreh, 2016; Wingfield, 2006), it is important to also document types of experiences these adolescents have in schools. This is especially true after 9/11 and various current sociopolitical contexts, such as the Arab Spring.

Ajrouch and Awad (2019) discussed three levels of discrimination that may be experienced by youth. The first level is individual discrimination, where one person treats another differently because of the other individual's membership in a social group (Benokraitis & Feagin, 1995). Examples include the use of racial epithets, such as "camel jockey" and "towel head," or calling someone a terrorist (Ajrouch & Awad, 2019). Individual discrimination can also be evident in social exclusion (Awad & Amayreh, 2016), where, for example, if peers hold negative stereotypes about Arabs, they might avoid interacting with their fellow peer and engage in bullying behaviors (Awad & Amayreh, 2016).

The second level is institutional/organizational discrimination (Ajrouch & Awad, 2019), which involves the practices and policies of institutions that have an unequal impact on specific individuals depending on their social group membership (Benokraitis & Feagin, 1995). An example of organizational discrimination includes the enforcement of policies that prohibit girls from wearing any head coverings in school (Ajrouch & Awad, 2019). Ajrouch and Awad (2019) note that because Islam and Arab identity is often conflated, anti-Muslim prejudice is often related to anti-Arab prejudice. An example in this case is the opposition to allowing major Muslim holidays to appear on public school district calendars (Ajrouch & Awad, 2019).

The third level is cultural discrimination (Ajrouch & Awad, 2019), which occurs when one group has the power to define pertinent cultural values for members of all social groups (Jones, 1997). Examples of cultural discrimination include the conceptions that tall and thin women who have blond hair and blue eyes are the epitome of beauty or that parenting styles in the West fostering independence from infancy are valued over parenting styles that foster interdependence on family (Ajrouch & Awad, 2019). Cultural discrimination can also be found in the media. For example, the absence of positive images of Arabs in American media combined with the multitude of adversarial images demonstrate the bias in depictions of Arabs to the American public, which essentially allows the negative images to resonate (Ajrouch & Awad, 2019).

Brenick, Schachner, Carvalheiro, and Karr (2019) identified the various types of prejudice and discrimination that can be found in the school system in particular. The authors speculate that prejudice and discrimination occurs in both overt and subtle forms, where overt is labeled as intentional and blatant and subtle is unintentional and ambiguous. Perceiving either of these forms of discrimination is equally impactful on minority youth development (Brenick et al., 2019). Brenick et al. (2019) further define these types under five categories: overt prejudice and discrimination, which may include verbal harassment and physical attacks based on the target's social group membership. Verbal harassment may include slurs, epithets, offensive jokes, and derogatory name-calling (Boysen, 2012).

Next, Brenick et al. (2019) mention the explicit and implicit discriminatory social exclusion by peers defined as relational bullying. Prejudice or biased-based bullying is seen as a more subtle form of prejudice by the social exclusion of minority peers (Brenick et al., 2019). Prime targets for this type of social exclusion are minorities who are culturally, linguistically, or ethnically diverse and hold a lower social status (Brenick et al., 2019; Hawley & Williford, 2015; Yeager, Fong, Lee, & Espelage, 2015).

The third category found in the school system is microaggressions (Brenick et al., 2019). Microaggressions are defined as the everyday slights, snubs, or exclusions that perpetrators often do not view as harmful or are completely unaware of their potential harm (Brenick et al., 2019; Sue, 2017). Examples of microaggressions against minorities include joking about their accents, excluding them or treating them as invisible, attributing a certain level of intelligence based on their ethnicity, and denying that their experiences of prejudice and discrimination exist (Brenick et al., 2019; Houshmand, Spanierman, & Tafarodi, 2014).

Discriminatory social exclusion may be considered as segregation in the school system, which leads to the fourth type of prejudice and discrimination: structural inequality and segregation (Brenick et al., 2019). Brenick et al. (2019) note that school segregation can be accepted from stakeholders within and outside the schools, including students, families, and communities. For example, research has shown that parents and communities have clearly demonstrated attitudes against inclusion and supporting segregation in school systems (Crowson & Brandes, 2010). Other means of structural inequality and segregation are through curriculum content and how it is presented (Brenick et al., 2019). Research shows that the majority of curricula exclude the perspectives, histories, and contributions of social minorities (Barrett, 2018). Brenick et al. (2019) call this implicit prejudice and discrimination by omitting diverse content or tokenizing minority groups by randomly or sporadically including them in the curriculum. This ultimately reinforces prejudiced social hierarchies by giving priority to certain groups (Brenick et al., 2019). What is even worse, the authors suggest, is when controversial and prejudiced views are explicitly presented in the curriculum (Brenick et al., 2019).

The final category presented is prejudice and discrimination exhibited by teachers (Brenick et al., 2019). Achievement expectations of teachers for minority students are often lower than their expectations for majority peers (Brenick et al., 2019). Research has shown that teachers often hold negative perceptions and implicit beliefs that minority students are not as teachable as their majority peers (Vervaet, D'Hondt, Van Houtte, & Stevens, 2016). Minority students are well aware of their teachers' views of them, which directly impacts their self-confidence, motivation, and performance levels (Brenick et al., 2019). Prejudice and discrimination are also evident in teachers' treatment and expectations of minority students pertaining to disciplinary action (Brenick et al., 2019). School staff often hold stereotypical expectations of minority youth viewing their behavior as aggressive and/or intentional and more deserving of disciplinary action (Brenick et al., 2019).

Arab American students have historically faced discrimination in the schools, especially after September 11, 2001 (Wingfield, 2006). The American Arab Anti-Discrimination Committee (ADC) publishes reports on discriminatory acts in the schools, documenting the most commonly occurring incidents as harassment, verbal abuse (i.e., derogatory names such as "towel head" and "camel jockey"), and the stereotyping of Arabs by students, teachers, and administrators (Ibish, 2001). Arab American students were associated with terrorism and incidents of political violence by other children (Ibish, 2001). These incidents occurred before 9/11; such incidents have increased ever since. Post-9/11 incidents are lucidly associated with the attacks and the war in Iraq (Ibish, 2008).

The American Arab Anti-Discrimination Committee (ADC) published a special report documenting incidents that occurred from the day of 9/11 through over a year later (Ibish, 2003). Hate crimes and discrimination were experienced by students of all ages, including kindergarten through college. Along with individual case stories, the report provided an overall picture of Arab American students' experiences in the schools:

> On September 11, and the days and weeks that followed, students reported physical assaults, death threats and overt ethnic and religious bigotry. Students were beaten, cursed, kicked, spat upon, and insulted. There were knife attacks, bomb threats, and vandalism. Many Muslim girls reported having their head covering pulled off. Teachers and other students made fun of their Arab names and made obscene and demeaning remarks. Students were harassed in classrooms, hallways, cafeterias and restrooms, on school buses and walking home from school. Sometimes teachers, administrators and coaches were more of a problem than the other students. Arab-American students, even young children in elementary school, were blamed for, or seen as being associated with, the attacks. A 5-year-old came home from school and asked her father, "What does it mean, terrorist? The other kids called me a terrorist." Some school officials actually went as far as calling the police or FBI to investigate students. (Ibish, 2003, p. 105)

Furthermore, Arab American Christians felt the need to wear Christian symbols conspicuously as to not be associated with their Muslim counterparts. Parent reports indicated that, due to these incidents, students were exhibiting "symptoms of stress, fear, tension, reluctance to go to school, bed-wetting, anger, and combativeness" (p. 106). One hundred and fifteen acts of physical violence, threats, harassment, and bias in the education system were reported in that year alone (Ibish, 2003). As time went by, reported incidents began to decrease but were still significantly more than before September 11, 2001 (Ibish, 2003).

A subsequent report by the ADC between the years 2003 and 2007 indicated an intensification in discrimination patterns in the 5 years following the attacks (Ibish, 2008). The report noted that the level of discrimination was clearly related to the 9/11 attacks, the "war on terrorism," and the Afghanistan and Iraq wars (p. 47). With such experiences, Arab American students were reportedly feeling higher levels of stress leading some to act out in anger (Ibish, 2008). Reports of incidents involved both students and teachers. Documented harassment by students involved physical assaults and confrontations, death threats, ethnic slurs and jokes, bullying, curses, mockery, and being spat on. Incidents by teachers involved assaults, ethnic and religious remarks, politicization of the classroom, attempts to discredit Islam or the Palestinian cause, associating Arab American or Muslim students and their families with terrorism, and allowing or fostering a negative atmosphere.

The latest report from the ADC (2011) stated a recent string of suicide deaths as a result of acts of discrimination and bullying in the K-12 system. The committee provided two case study examples.

> A third grade Arab-American student was humiliated in front of his classmates after his teacher referred to him as the "next terrorist." This resulted in the bullying of the student by his classmates. The parents of the child immediately noticed that something was wrong. After explaining to his parents what had happened, they immediately called the ADC for assistance. The school administration took immediate action and fired the teacher… (p. 6)
>
> A concerned Arab-American father has very recently contacted ADC about an incident that occurred with the high school son, who is part of a sporting team. The son received an invitation letter from his teammates to a private event. The letter stated that "no Arabs are allowed at the event." Upon further investigation, a teacher seems to have taken part in drafting the invite during school hours on school grounds… (p. 6)

A more recent incident was seen in 2015 with a student, Ahmed Mohamed, in Texas who was arrested at school for bringing in a homemade clock that his teacher assumed was a bomb (Selk, 2015). Society seemed split on whether the teacher and the authorities were justified in their actions or if this was an incident of racial profiling. There was question whether their biases against Arabs were motivations in their reactions to this child.

Making matters more complicated is the fact that the Arab culture is rarely included in the multicultural paradigm in schools (Abu El-Haj, 2006; Britto, 2008; Schwartz, 1999; Seikaly, 2001; Wingfield, 2006). This in and of itself may be considered a form of discrimination by ignoring that this culture exists (Suleiman, 2000). According to Schwartz (1999) and Suleiman (1996), schools historically have not actively acknowledged Arab culture or tried to counteract stereotyping against Arabs. Prior to the terrorist attacks of 9/11, Arab communities were defined as racially and ethnically "invisible" by Arab American scholars (Naber, 2008). It was not until after the attacks that Arab cultures began to be added to the multicultural paradigm in academics and popular discussions (Naber, 2008). The attacks of 9/11 were the catalyst for educators to take action against these issues (Wingfield, 2006).

Even so, since 9/11, researchers report that low tolerance of Arab American students continues to be evident by the increased incidences of bullying and discrimination in the school environment (Abu El-Haj & Bonet, 2011; Britto, 2008; Haboush & Alyan, 2016). The problem with the inclusion of Arab culture and history in the curriculum of public schools is twofold: it is insignificant or nonexistent in many situations yet, when present, it often contains inaccurate information (Wingfield, 2006). This absence and misinformation result in Arab youth feeling alienated and misrecognized in their schools (Abu El-Haj, 2006; Suleiman, 2004). Abu El-Haj (2006) calls for the creation of "just, responsive educational environments for Arab American youth" (p. 15) and states that "educators must move beyond a model of cultural understanding and attend, instead, to the particular processes of racial subordination to which these youths are subjected within and outside of school" (p. 15).

Few studies have directly explored self-reported school experiences of Arab American adolescents. Tabbah (2016)[1] shed some light on this issue using a survey study for which students were asked to report on their experiences of discrimination in school and provide details about their experiences. The study served to explore and describe specific experiences and perceptions of inclusion and accuracy of the Arab American culture in the multicultural paradigm in school through the voices of Arab American youth. Both individual and group experiences were obtained. This exploratory study sought to answer the following questions: (a) What types of experiences are evident from the reports of this sample? (b) What is the frequency of inclusion of the Arab American culture reported? (c) What themes are evident from students' reports on accuracy of information provided in the multicultural paradigm regarding the Arab American culture?

Tabbah (2016) reported that 240 surveys were distributed to subjects who volunteered to participate in the study. Sixty-eight students returned the surveys (28.3% response rate); two students did not meet the eligibility criteria for age, one student attended home school, and four students did not fully complete the forms. Thus, there were 61 valid respondents between the ages of 12 and 18 years. The average age of the 61 respondents was 15.3 years. Forty-five (73.8%) of the respondents were in high school. There were 28 males (45.9%) and 33 females (54.1%). Students were predominately Muslim (51, 83.6%). Christians comprised 14.8% (9) of the sample, and one person reported no religious affiliation (1.6%). The majority of the participants resided in the Midwestern region of the United States. Two-thirds of the students (67.2%) were first-generation Americans. Ancestry included Palestinian (34.4%), Syrian (23.0%), mixed Arab ancestry (28%), Egyptian (4.9%), Iraqi (4.9%), Jordanian (3.3%), and Yemeni (1.6%).

Due to the fact that there were no established instruments that addressed specific concerns relative to this study, Tabbah (2016) developed a questionnaire to obtain

[1] Reprinted by permission from *Journal for Multicultural Education* (2016), 10(4), 449–464. ©2016 Emerald Group Publishing Limited https://www.emerald.com/insight/content/doi/10.1108/JME-05-2015-0014/full/html. Authors retain rights to reuse work in future works through Emerald Group Publishing Limited https://www.emeraldgrouppublishing.com/services/authors/author-policies/author-rights

details of experiences with discrimination. Participants were asked the following two questions: (1) "Prejudice and discrimination is when people treat other people badly and/or differently because of their ethnicity, race, gender, religion or other things. Has anyone treated you badly or differently in your school because of your ethnicity or being Arab American? Please circle one. Yes or No. If yes, please describe what happened." (2) "Now think about other people who are close to you in your life. Has someone close to you ever been treated badly or differently in their school because of their ethnicity or being Arab American? Please circle one. Yes or No. If yes, please describe what happened." Students were asked to elaborate on their experiences for a qualitative review. To gather perceptions of curricular inclusion, students were asked: "Does your school teach about the Arab American culture either in your classes or through events like cultural awareness week? Please circle yes or no. If you circled yes, do you think that what is taught about the Arab culture is right or true? Please circle yes or no. If you circled no, can you tell me what they teach about the culture that is wrong?" The data from the open-ended questions were analyzed for specific types of experiences in the schools and perceptions of curricular inclusion and accuracy of Arab American culture and history. A demographic questionnaire was also included to gather data on age, gender, religion, and ancestry.

A survey research design was used in attempt to obtain samples from this population throughout the country. Because Arab American students were difficult to identify and schools were reluctant to single-out populations for studies, Tabbah (2016) used a non-random, convenience sample. A snowball sampling method—a technique where each person or group contacted was instructed to contact other potential participants—was used to recruit participants (Vogt, 2005). Snowball sampling began by contacting Arab American organizations around the country by email and phone, six of which expressed interest in helping recruit participants. The organizations included Arab American Family Services in Illinois, the Center for Arabic Culture in Massachusetts, the Alif Institute in Georgia, the Noor Islamic Cultural Center in Ohio, the Islamic Center of Cleveland in Ohio, and the Alif Ba Arabic Learning Center in Ohio. Four of these organizations sent letters that described the study and provided the author's contact information to their members. Interested participants contacted the author by email and provided a mailing address for which to send the surveys. The Noor Islamic Cultural Center and the Islamic Center of Cleveland asked the author to attend their youth group sessions to meet with and recruit participants. Interested participants in this scenario were provided with pre-paid survey packets to complete and mail back to the author. To be eligible for inclusion in the study, participants needed to (a) self-identify as an Arab American, (b) be between the ages of 12 and 18 years, and (c) be enrolled in a public or private school in the United States.

Students were asked to describe their experiences of being treated differently in the schools due to their ethnicity. A little over half of the sample (50.8%) reported being treated differently or negatively personally, vicariously, or both. Experiences were examined from the reports and coded into categories as follows. Experiences involving name-calling (e.g., terrorist, camel jockey, towelhead), the excessive use of language to intentionally annoy, insult or humiliate another and experiences involving physical harm or use of physical means to taunt or humiliate another were defined as bullying/harassment. Experiences defined as stereotyping of Arabs involved statements from others where both racial and religious stereotypes were explicit or implied. Stereotypes identified included both religious and ethnic/racial.

Twenty-four students personally experienced being treated negatively or differently at school. These experiences overwhelmingly involved bullying/harassment by peers. Intertwined in these experiences were notes of racial and religious stereotyping of Arabs. Many of the students' reports contained multiple themes of stereotypes. Pseudonyms for participants will be used throughout this section. Two students described being racially and religiously stereotyped in general and feeling an overall sense of hatred for Arabs from the majority. Hints of stereotyping Islam with fanaticism were noted by Omar (second quote below):

> Except for one time when a girl told me she hated Arabs because of me, most instances haven't been direct, just implied. Some people assume that I was poor and we ate on the ground in Syria. Some aren't disrespectful to me in particular, but have a general distaste for the Arab ethnicity. A lot of people harness a hatred for the Middle East, saying things like "let's just bomb the whole place!"
>
> People automatically think I'm a dirty person (no hygiene). They think I'm pretty radical when it comes to religious values.

Ahmed described experiences with bullying/harassment because of his ethnicity during the time of 9/11 specifically:

> Though I am a teen now, I was in a public elementary school during the time of nine/eleven. At that time, I was constantly insulted, picked on, beat up, and got things such as trash and food thrown at me. Things aren't as bad now as they were but discrimination is still everywhere.

Six students specifically reported being called a terrorist, three of which provided incidents of classmates referencing bombs. Maya described an incident where she was taunted by another student claiming that she was a terrorist. Translations for Arabic transliterations are provided in brackets:

> I have been called a terrorist on many occasions since 9/11. Especially since I wear the hijab [head cover], I have heard comments such as "she is a woman terrorist who is hiding a bomb under her hijab." In fact, during my sophomore year when I ran for class president, an opposing campaign said, "Don't vote for a female terrorist as a class president- she'll blow you up with the bomb she is hiding under her hijab!"

Similarly, Shireen described being verbally harassed and stereotyped as a terrorist by a fellow classmate. This student in particular also reported feeling that certain staff hold religious and racial biases against Arab students:

> A girl in my class was divided up in teams in countries and she was on a Arabic team. When she found out she said, "Hey Shireen, I'm on a terrorist team" and kept repeating it until I got mad. Another story is our librarian in our school treats Americans a lot better than Muslims and other of my Arabic friends.

In addition to bomb references, two students reported being referred to as unintelligent and the effects this has had on them:

> Sometimes people would say "you're a stupid Arab" and I would just ignore. Other times they would say that I'm going to bomb the school. Some people would joke around and say some of that but it still hurt my feelings.
>
> People call me a stupid Arab. Also people call me a terrorist because of 911 which I don't like.

Rayan, a Christian student described his experience with the specific stereotype of Arabs being Muslim. He reported:

> Some kids found out I was Arab so they called me Mohammad (even though I'm, Christian) for one months until I told my head master.

Another theme of religious and racial bias that arose was female Muslim students being treated differently because of the way they dress with the hijab, or head covering. For example, Sara discussed how the way she acts and dresses conveys that she is an Arab Muslim and how this attracts verbal insults and bullying/harassment from classmates:

> I express myself with the way I dress and act. When people see this, they can tell I am Arab and may call me a terrorist, not talk to me, or make fun of the way I look. I don't let this bother me but it would make me feel better if I was treated normally.

Sometimes students seemed to be left with confusion and hurtful feelings after experiences. For example, Moussa was confused as to why another student told him to go back to where he came from. This experience gives an example of how Arab American students may be perceived and treated as the "other," as described in the literature:

> This rarely happens, once there was this kid mad at me. I don't really know why. He told me to go back to where I came from. It didn't make any sense because I was born and raised here. I just get so annoyed and mad because they don't know me, who are they to say that to me? I hate the fact that it gets to me and for the rest of the day I just feel so horrible inside.

Another example of otherness may be implied in Layla's reports of lack of friendship when she was younger due to being Arab:

> People in my school use the term towel heads and terrorist. And when I was younger no one wanted to be my friend because of my race, they also bullied me after Sept. 11th.

Zayna spoke to her peers' lack of understanding of certain aspects of her culture and referred to questions asked by them to clarify her customs:

> I've had someone call me a terrorist, but he stopped. People make fun of me for not eating pork, but really, I don't care. A lot of people ask me questions about my religion and ethnicity and are truly interested. Others, wonder why I don't date or why I don't dress the same, even though I don't wear a veil. They just wonder why I don't wear short shorts and stuff like that.

Twenty-two students reported that they knew someone close to them with negative experiences or witnessed another individual being treated negatively due to their ethnicity. Experiences were similarly categorized under bullying/harassment, racial stereotyping, and religious stereotyping. Reports were similar to personal experiences reported in that they largely involved bullying/harassment with notes of religious and racial stereotyping.

Several students reported knowing of other students who were bullied/harassed because of their accents and limited English proficiency. Faysa described a young boy who experiences verbal abuse due to his accent:

> They make fun of a young Syrian boy, age of 9. He has a strong accent when he speaks English, so the children make fun of him. They tease him very much.

Saeed reported on a boy who avoids talking due to fear of being made fun of because of the way he speaks:

> One time there was a boy named Farooq, and he came from Jordan, and he only knew a couple English words. There were some kids who were his friends, and some kids made fun of him b/c of the way he talks, and now he doesn't talk a lot.

Nadine, a female adolescent who moved to the country only 1 year ago, described her friends' experiences with bullying/harassment after recently moving to the U.S. as well:

> Some of my friends get bullied b/c of their English. I learned English before I came to the USA but I still have an accent though. My friend just started to learn English when they came here so they get picked on and cursed at for the lack of their English and b/c people know for sure my friends are not going to understand it.

Two students reported knowing of Arab friends being physically assaulted or harassed by peers on school grounds. Sami described a physical fight that occurred after his friend tried to defend his religion:

> One of my friends from another school was fighting another person who was talking badly about Islam. Many of this person's friends were physically hurting my friend until teachers tried to split up the conflict but by then my friend had already been knocked unconscious by a kick in the head while he was lying on the ground.

Amal, an Arab Muslim student, spoke specifically about her friends' experiences with bullying, and she cited an example of her sibling's experience in the classroom with a teacher implying religious stereotypes:

> Once a teacher told my sisters class that she didn't feel safe flying on an airplane when Muslims are there.

Similar to personal experiences, a theme of religious and racial bias that arose was female Muslim students being treated differently because of the way they dress with the hijab. Noora, who attended a private Islamic school, described her female Muslim friends' experiences in the public school system with bullying/harassment:

> A few of my friends who wear hijab have had it pulled off in hallways. They tell me about the dirty looks they get. All of these friends go to public school. None of my private school friends (even if it's my school) don't have these kinds of problems.

Two additional students expressed the evident distinction of how Arab Muslim women wearing the hijab are treated as compared to women who do not cover. Dania particularly noted the equation of society automatically seeing her as Arab once she decides to wear the hijab:

> For me since I still haven't put on the hijab, people don't know I am Arab until I tell them. But most of my close friends and relatives do wear the hijab so others can tell they are Muslims. People make fun of them, but I feel the ones that do make fun of them by saying lame bomb jokes, don't know what they are saying but instead are saying what they are taught/see on the American news.

In terms of inclusion of the Arab culture in the multicultural paradigm at school, 59 students answered the question. The majority of the sample ($n = 36$) reported that their school did not include Arabs in the multicultural curriculum. From students who reported that their school did include Arabs in curriculum ($n = 23$), six reported that the teachings of the culture were inaccurate. The themes that arose from these reports included the misconception that all Arabs are Muslim:

> I think that most of what they teach is right and true but the overall impression they give is that it is all Islamic and that it's not a whole lot of fun. While the Middle Eastern majority is Muslim, there are a lot of Christians there, and the churches are beautiful. Easter and Christmas are bigger in Syria than they are here.

Three students specifically expressed the misinformation about beliefs of the Islamic faith when taught about the Arab culture. Two students spoke of the stereotypes and misconceptions of the role of women in the culture. Hazem reported:

> Sometimes they say "arranged marriage", forced to wear hijab, women aren't treated fairly.

Two students expressed their frustration with biases and misinformation they found apparent in their schools when it comes to their culture in the curriculum. Sumayah (second quotation below) expressed the biases in school policy when it came to students of different cultures expressing themselves in clothing. Translations of Arabic transliterations are provided in brackets:

> They don't teach anything. Everything and anything they talk to us about that includes Araby [Arabic] is always negative. They always say we killed this or bombed this but they never show how many Middle Eastern people die every day. I hate this subject cuz u know everyone is look at you and thinkin all those things…Yes I am proud of what I am but sometimes I get so frustrated because I thought there was a separation between church and state. But they always bring up Islam as it its wrong…I have a history teacher who I will ask a question and he will avoid answering it. And its not just me it 3 other students yes (Muslim) students. We're the only ones in the class. I just feel that if there is not going to tell the truth then the subject should not be brought up… Also they never teach about the culture, its either Black History month or something else the only time the middle east in mentioned is with 3 things "oil, war, 9/11" that's it. Not once do you hear about our food, music, traditions, or why we fast or what Eid [holiday] is or anything. But yet Christmas is celebrated and thanksgiving are and we get off but yet there hallmark holidays? What's that about. And we get marked absent for take (emphasized 1) day off for Eid [holiday]? And some of us who only miss that can lose the attendance award I think thats not fair. But again lifes not fair I guess…
>
> One time when we were learning about Rome we had to learn about the Christianity, and there were Bible teachings, but we have to skip the lesson about ancient Arabia and the teachings of Muhammad but we have to learn about Christianity. School bias against Arab (Moslem) children a boy was given detention for wearing a shirt with the wording (Allah) and sent home. But another student was with attire of same with (I love Jesus) seen in school all day (no reprimand on this student).

Policies similar to those reported imply to students that one culture or belief is superior to the other; one practice is punishable while the other is not. Since youth look to their elders for model behaviors, these types of acts may send a message to youth that this behavior is acceptable. Such forms of bias can surely single out students and make them feel "othered." This may also create a sense of disconnect and confusion for students in terms of identity development and who they are as an individual. For example, what they learn about their culture at home is positive while what they learn about their culture in school is negative, and they are punished for expressing their culture/beliefs in school.

Tabbah (2016) sought to explore and present real-time experiences of a sample of Arab American adolescents and their perceptions of inclusion in the multicultural paradigm in their schools. Experiences reported both personally and vicariously were categorized as bullying/harassment, racial stereotypes, and religious stereotypes. The experiences were largely considered bullying/harassment combined with biases and behaviors involved with racial and religious stereotypes. For some reports, racial and religious stereotypes went hand-in-hand, and it was difficult to separate the two constructs. This difficulty stems from the intertwining of the concepts of Arab and Muslim evident in student reports. For example, for reports of students being called a terrorist, it is not clear whether this is more racially or religiously charged or perhaps equally charged by biases from peers. Themes that arose in their reports of experiences both personally and vicariously include the stereotypes of Arabs being Muslims, being terrorists, and bombing. Students were faced with these labels and generalized into these categories. Themes of being treated as "other" were also noted in students' experiences as well as a lack of understanding of aspects of the culture. Arab Muslim female students wearing the hijab have an additional burden to bear as they become more "visible" when they cover their hair, which appears to make them more susceptible to these experiences. One student made a reference to individuals acting the way they do because of what they are taught and what they see in the media, which leads back to cultural conditioning and the importance of challenging cultural misconceptions in society.

Additionally, over half of the sample reported that their school does not include the Arab American culture in the multicultural paradigm. Of the 23 students reporting that the culture was included, six of them provided details of inaccuracies in the curricula including stereotypical teachings of religion, Arab women, and general aspects of the culture. Frustrations were noted with the lack of focus on the positive aspects of the culture including traditions, foods, music, and history. Students also noted double-standards in school policy, especially in terms of cultural and religious expressions.

A recent study by Kumar, Karabenick, Warnke, Hany, and Seay (2019) examined the school experiences of Arab/Arab American, Chaldean, African American, and European American students, including interactions with teachers and peers, the curriculum, and school policies. The authors used an exploratory mixed methods design with two phases where phase 1 used a qualitative design and phase 2 used a quantitative design. Phase 1 included the use of focus groups to obtain data on the experiences of students, while phase 2 used the data from phase 1 to develop a measure called culturally inclusive and responsive curricular learning environments. For the purposes of this chapter, only details regarding phase 1 of the study are discussed.

The study sample was taken from 12 middle schools in two districts, which had significant immigrant populations and neighborhoods that were characterized as ethnic enclaves for Arab/Arab American immigrants. Seven schools made up the first school district where Arab/Arab American students were a significant portion of the student body ranging from a predominant majority of over 90% to a minority of under 5%. In the second district, Arab/Arab American students were nonexistent. The focus group sample was comprised of 333 eighth-grade adolescents (144 Arab/Arab American, 41 Chaldean, 48 African American, and 100 European American). The students participated in one of 57 focus group sessions (24 Arab/Arab American, 8 Chaldean, 7 African American, and 18 European American), which averaged six students per interview. The authors systematically selected participants based on random sampling of eighth-grade students, stratified by ethnicity and primary language spoken at home as noted in school records. Due to the fact that the census identifies people of Middle Eastern origin as white, the authors further stratified whites by language spoken at home to distinguish Chaldean and Arab/Arab American students from their European American peers. The focus groups were ethnically homogenous in order to provide a safe space in which participants could discuss openly issues related to their shared social identities within the school setting. Focus group interviews took place on school property and lasted about 45 min each. Questions asked during the interviews sought to obtain student perceptions regarding composition of groups and permeability of groups and intergroup conflict, cultural sensitivity of schools and teachers, and curriculum and school policies. Discussion of results will focus on the Arab/Arab American sample.

Results from thematic analyses of both individual and group levels revealed four main themes from student perceptions and experiences of their schools' cultural responsiveness. The first theme was perceptions of teachers as prejudiced and culturally insensitive versus respectful and culturally responsive. Teachers were either perceived as culturally responsive and demonstrating authenticity, respect for, and openness to cultural differences among students, or perceived as prejudice and insensitive to these differences. This was found explicitly with Arab/Arab American, Chaldean, and African American students. Results among Arab American and Chaldean students revealed perceptions that teachers did not like Arabs or Chaldeans. Negative perceptions of teachers focused on their perceived biases toward Arab and Chaldean students' ethnic and/or religious differences. Interviews revealed students' frustrations with teachers being prejudice and perpetuating stereotypes about Arab and Chaldean communities. Where Arab and Chaldean students were a minority in school, they reported concern regarding teachers' personal biases on sensitive issues of Middle Eastern geopolitics. Teachers would shut down opportunities for students to express their opinions, perspectives, and concerns regarding their culturally situated experiences and dismiss issues related to students' lives.

Arab American students in ethnic enclave schools reported more positive experiences and described culturally responsive teachers as oriented toward cultural openness and having respect for differences. A common theme within cultural responsiveness was teachers having authenticity and care for their students regardless of differences. Teachers who showed cultural respect and openness facilitated opportunities for intercultural dialogue, and their classrooms were perceived as safe spaces for these students to openly discuss and express their opinions regarding important world issues.

The second theme that emerged was culturally responsive and inclusive classroom curriculum. The authors found differences in perceptions of the curriculum based on different identity groups and the proximal majority/minority status of students in the various schools. In general, Arab/Arab American students agreed that the curriculum was not inclusive, especially when it came to social studies and language arts. However, in schools that were predominantly Arab, the students reported more positive experiences with culturally responsive curricula, including the use of inclusive literature and the opportunity to study Arabic as an elective language. Arab/Arab American students in non-ethnic enclave schools reported an absence of cultural representation in classroom curricula and feelings of exclusion related to this absence. These students were required to attend outside activities within their own ethnic community to learn about their history, culture, and language. They reported feeling that their teachers and administrators did not care that they wanted to learn more about their own cultural history in school.

The third theme involved intergroup relationships in schools. Interviews revealed that the cultural and ethnic composition of the student body was an important factor in defining in-group and intergroup relationships and intercultural understanding. In more homogenous schools, the majority of students reported that school was like a second home to them, and intergroup relationships were positive. In schools where Arab/Arab American students were the minority, their participation in extracurricular activities provided them opportunities to develop cross-group relationships and enhanced their sense of belonging. However, these students frequently reported experiences of discrimination and prejudice in their schools. One of the most commonly reported discriminatory acts among peers was name calling. For example, where European American students were a majority, the label "terrorist" caused great distress among Arab/Arab American students.

The fourth and final theme found was perceptions of school policies and practices. Schools that were considered ethnic enclaves for Arab/Arab American students enforced culturally responsive practices and policies designed to ensure educational access for Arab/Arab American and immigrant students. These policies and practices were inclusive of students' cultural and religious backgrounds such as observing religious holidays and food restrictions. Conversely, schools where Arab/Arab American students were minorities were perceived as unwelcoming. Further, when students in these schools were asked what the schools could do to be more culturally responsive, they often answered cynically with statements such as "Can't do anything," "they don't care," and feelings of exclusion from peers "Cause they (European American peers) don't understand us…What's normal to them is not normal to us; what's normal to us is not normal to them…People stay with their own kind…It's hard to be with someone who doesn't understand you" (p. 98). Students suggested that schools and classrooms should be safe spaces by allowing more opportunities for open and reasonable discussion to promote intercultural understanding.

In conclusion, Kumar et al. (2019) indicated that results from their study showed that cultural responsiveness in the school context encompasses all aspects of the environment, including school policies and practice, teacher attitudes and beliefs regarding culturally diverse students, and intergroup relationships with peers. Alienation, marginalization, and invisibility in the school environment were common themes through the focus group interviews. Arab/Arab American students felt particularly vulnerable and discriminated against. Participants called on teachers and peers to engage in activities to promote cultural competence and sensitivity (Kumar et al., 2019).

Conclusion

The literature demonstrates that stereotypes, misconceptions, and discrimination from general society has infiltrated the school systems in America for Arab youth. These issues were evident prior to 9/11 but became magnified after the terrorist attacks. The attacks served as an impetus to increase awareness and knowledge regarding Arab cultures due to the amplification of misconceptions and discrimination experiences of Arab Americans. Educators and researchers began to take action in this endeavor. While the research on experiences of Arab youth in the school system is scarce, it is growing compared to the pre-9/11 era. The research currently available shows that discrimination is evident throughout all facets of the school environment, including practice and policy and relationships with staff and peers. In terms of relationships, lack of cultural understanding on behalf of school staff and peers is clear. In addition, misrepresentation and/or lack of representation in multicultural curricula is evidently a major issue throughout the literature presented. Given the history of experiences with discrimination, Arab American youth may be at-risk of developmental growth (Al-Hazza & Bucher, 2010; Suleiman, 1996; Wingfield, 2006; Wingfield & Karaman, 2009).

References

Abu El-Haj, T. R. (2006). Race, politics, and Arab American youth: Shifting frameworks for conceptualizing educational equity. *Educational Policy, 20*, 13–34. https://doi.org/10.1177/0895904805285287.

Abu El-Haj, T. R., & Bonet, S. W. (2011). Education, citizenship, and the politics of belonging: Youth from Muslim transnational communities and the "war on terror". *Review of Research in Education, 35*(1), 29–59. https://doi.org/10.3102/0091732x10383209.

ADC. (2011). *The 2010 ADC legal report: Legal advocacy and policy review*. Washington, DC: American Arab Anti-Discrimination Committee.

Ajrouch, K. J., & Awad, G. H. (2019). An ecological approach to childhood prejudice: The case of Arab Americans. In H. E. Fitzgerald, D. J. Johnson, D. B. Qin, F. A. Villarruel, & J. Norder (Eds.), *Handbook of children and prejudice: Integrating research, practice, and policy* (pp. 147–159). Cham, Switzerland: Springer.

Al-Hazza, T., & Bucher, K. T. (2010). Bridging a cultural divide with literature about Arabs and Arab Americans. *Middle School Journal, 41*, 4–11. https://doi.org/10.2307/23047567.

Al-Khatab, A. (1999). Search of equity for Arab-American students in public schools of the United States. *Education, 120*(2), 254.

Asi, M., & Beaulieu, D. (2013). *Arab households in the United States: 2006–2010.* Retrieved September 10, 2019, from https://www.census.gov/library/publications/2013/acs/acsbr10-20.html

Awad, G. H., & Amayreh, W. M. (2016). Discrimination: Heightened prejudice post 9/11 and psychological outcomes. In M. M. Amer & G. H. Awad (Eds.), *Handbook of Arab American psychology* (pp. 63–75). New York: Routledge.

Banks, J. A. (2009). *Teaching strategies for ethnic studies* (8th ed.). Boston, MA: Allyn and Bacon.

Barrett, M. (2018). How schools can promote the intercultural competence of young people. *European Psychologist, 23*(1), 93–104. https://doi.org/10.1027/1016-9040/a000308.

Benokraitis, N. V., & Feagin, J. R. (1995). *Modern sexism: Blatant, subtle, and covert discrimination* (2nd ed.). Englewood Cliffs, NJ: Prentice Hall.

Boysen, G. A. (2012). Teacher and student perceptions of microaggressions in college classrooms. *College Teaching, 60*, 122–129.

Brenick, A., Schachner, M. K., Carvalheiro, D., & Karr, E. (2019). (No) space for prejudice! Varied forms of negative outgroup attitudes and ethnic discrimination and how they develop or can be prevented in the classroom. In H. E. Fitzgerald, D. J. Johnson, D. B. Qin, F. A. Villarruel, & J. Norder (Eds.), *Handbook of children and prejudice: Integrating research, practice, and policy* (pp. 315–330). Cham, Switzerland: Springer.

Britto, P. R. (2008). Who am I? Ethnic identity formation of Arab Muslim children in contemporary U.S. society. *Journal of American Academy of Child and Adolescent Psychiatry, 47*(8), 853–857.

Crowson, H. M., & Brandes, J. A. (2010). Predicting community opposition to inclusion in schools: The role of social dominance, contact, intergroup anxiety, and economic conservatism. *The Journal of Psychology, 144*(2), 121–144. https://doi.org/10.1080/00223980903472151.

Haboush, K. L., & Alyan, H. (2016). School psychology: Enhancing school climate and school connectedness. In M. M. Amer & G. H. Awad (Eds.), *Handbook of Arab American psychology* (pp. 318–330). New York: Routledge.

Hawley, P. H., & Williford, A. (2015). Articulating the theory of bullying intervention programs: Views from social psychology, social work, and organizational science. *Journal of Applied Developmental Psychology, 37*, 3–15. https://doi.org/10.1016/j.appdev.2014.11.006.

Houshmand, S., Spanierman, L. B., & Tafarodi, R. W. (2014). Excluded and avoided: Racial microaggressions targeting Asian international students in Canada. *Cultural Diversity and Ethnic Minority Psychology, 20*, 377–388. https://doi.org/10.1037/a0035404.

Ibish, H. E. (2001). *Report on hate crimes and discrimination against Arab Americans 1998–2000.* Washington, DC: American Arab Anti-Discrimination Committee Research Institute.

Ibish, H. E. (2003). *Report on hate crimes and discrimination against Arab Americans: The post-September 11 Backlash September 11, 2001 - October 11, 2002.* Washington, DC: American Arab Anti-Discrimination Committee Research Institute.

Ibish, H. E. (2008). *Report on hate crimes and discrimination against Arab Americans 2003–2007.* Washington, DC: American Arab Anti-Discrimination Committee Research Institute.

Jones, J. M. (1997). *Prejudice and racism* (2nd ed.). New York: McGraw-Hill.

Kumar, R., Karabenick, S. A., Warnke, J. H., Hany, S., & Seay, N. (2019). Culturally inclusive and responsive curricular learning environments (CIRCLEs): An exploratory sequential mixed-methods approach. *Contemporary Educational Psychology, 57*, 87–105. https://doi.org/10.1016/j.cedpsych.2018.10.005.

Naber, N. (2008). Introduction: Arab Americans and U.S. racial formations. In A. Jamal & N. Naber (Eds.), *Race and Arab Americans before and after 9/11* (pp. 1–45). Syracuse, NY: Syracuse University Press.

Nieto, S. (1996). *Affirming diversity: The sociopolitical context of multicultural education* (2nd ed.). New York: Longman.

Nieto, S. (2000). *Affirming diversity: The sociopolitical context of multicultural education* (3rd ed.). White Plains, NY: Longman.

Schwartz, W. (1999). *Arab American students in public schools*. New York: ERIC Clearinghouse on Urban Education.

Seikaly, Z. A. (2001). At risk of prejudice: The Arab American community. *Social Education, 65*, 349–351. Retrieved from http://www.socialstudies.org/system/files/publications/se/6506/650604.html.

Selk, A. (2015). Ahmed Mohamed swept up, 'hoax bomb' charges swept away as Irving teen's story floods social media. *The Dallas Morning News*. Retrieved from http://www.dallasnews.com/news/community-news/northwest-dallas-county/headlines/20150915-irving-ninth-grader-arrested-after-taking-homemade-clock-to-school.ece

Sue, D. W. (2017). Microaggressions and "evidence": Empirical or experiential reality? *Perspectives on Psychological Science, 12*(1), 170–172. https://doi.org/10.1177/1745691616664437.

Suleiman, M. F. (1996). *Educating the Arab American child: Implications for teachers*. Retrieved from http://eric.ed.gov/?id=ED392864

Suleiman, M. F. (2000). *Teaching about Arab Americans: What social studies teachers should know*. Retrieved from http://eric.ed.gov/?id=ED442714

Suleiman, M. F. (2001a). *Image making of Arab Americans: Implications for teachers in diverse settings*. Retrieved from http://eric.ed.gov/?id=ED452310

Suleiman, M. F. (2001b). *Image making of Arab Americans: Implications for teachers in diverse settings*. Paper presented at the California Association for Bilingual Education Conference, Los Angeles, CA.

Suleiman, M. F. (2004). Image making and invisible minorities: A case of Arab American students. In G. S. Goodman & K. Carey (Eds.), *Critical multicultural conversations* (pp. 79–91). Cresskill, NJ: Hampton.

Tabbah, R. (2016). The perils of Arab American adolescents post 9/11. *Journal for Multicultural Education, 10*(4), 449–464. https://doi.org/10.1108/JME-05-2015-0014.

Vervaet, R., D'Hondt, F., Van Houtte, M., & Stevens, P. A. (2016). The ethnic prejudice of Flemish teachers: The role of ethnic school composition and of teachability. *Cultural Diversity and Ethnic Minority Psychology, 22*(4), 552–562. https://doi.org/10.1037/cdp0000085.

Vogt, W. P. (2005). *Dictionary of statistics and methodology* (3rd ed.). Thousand Oaks, CA: Sage.

Wingfield, M. (2006). Arab Americans: Into the multicultural mainstream. *Equity & Excellence in Education, 39*, 253–266. https://doi.org/10.1080/10665680600788453.

Wingfield, M., & Karaman, B. (2009). *Arab stereotypes and American educators*. Retrieved June 10, 2019, from https://www.adc.org/arab-stereotypes-and-american-educators/

Yeager, D. S., Fong, C. J., Lee, H. Y., & Espelage, D. L. (2015). Declines in efficacy of anti-bullying programs among older adolescents: Theory and a three-level meta-analysis. *Journal of Applied Developmental Psychology, 37*, 36–51. https://doi.org/10.1016/j.appdev.2014.11.005.

Developmental Theories Relevant to Arab American Youth

Introduction

Discrimination has been found to influence various developmental outcomes. During adolescence, individuals have developed the cognitive capacities—both intellectual and social knowledge regarding group membership and understanding of cultural stereotypes—to experience and recognize multiple forms of racial and ethnic discrimination (Benner & Graham, 2013). Before discussing the research found regarding the outcomes in Arab American adolescents, it is important to discuss the developmental processes and the theories that exist pertaining to development and discrimination. Several theories exist regarding the effects of discrimination on development, including identity, self-concept, and general well-being. The existing research regarding Arab Americans is based on the theories outlined below. This chapter presents the various theories that are most relevant to Arab American youth. Developmental processes in adolescence are discussed in detail along with how discrimination has been found to affect these processes. The dialogue sets the stage for why and how discrimination in various settings, including the school system, influences critical aspects of development in minority youth.

Bronfenbrenner's Ecology of Human Development

Bronfenbrenner proposed that human development is related to a multi-person systems of interaction and, in terms of examination, requires that various aspects of the environment be taken into consideration beyond the immediate one involving the individual (Bronfenbrenner, 1977). Bronfenbrenner (1977) coined this scientific perspective as the "ecology of human development" (p. 514) and defined it as:

> the scientific study of the progressive, mutual accommodation, throughout the life span, between a growing human organism and the changing immediate environments in which it

R. Tabbah, *Arab American Youth*, Advancing Responsible Adolescent Development, https://doi.org/10.1007/978-3-030-66804-4_6

lives, as this process is affected by relations obtaining within and between these immediate settings, as well as the larger social contexts, both formal and informal, in which the settings are embedded. (p. 514)

Bronfenbrenner (1977) further defined the environment as an ecological environment that "is conceived topologically as a nested arrangement of structures, each contained within the next" (p. 514). The ecological environment consists of four successive levels: microsystem, mesosystem, exosystem, and macrosystem (Bronfenbrenner, 1977). Bronfenbrenner (1977) provided the following definitions for each level:

- A microsystem is the complex of relations between the developing person and environment in an immediate setting containing that person (e.g., home, school, workplace, etc.). A setting is defined as a place with particular physical features in which the participants engage in particular activities in particular roles (e.g., daughter, parent, teacher, employee, etc.) for particular periods of time. The factors of place, time, physical features, activity, participant, and role constitute the elements of a setting. (p. 514)
- A mesosystem comprises the interrelations among major settings containing the developing person at a particular point in his or her life. Thus, for an American 12-year-old, the mesosystem typically encompasses interactions among family, school, and peer group; for some children, it might also include church, camp, or workplace, although the last would be less common in the United States than in some other societies. In sum, stated succinctly, a mesosystem is a system of microsystems. (p. 515)
- An exosystem is an extension of the mesosystem embracing other specific social structures, both formal and informal, that do not themselves contain the developing person but impinge upon or encompass the immediate settings in which that person is found, and thereby influence, delimit, or even determine what goes on there. These structures include the major institutions of the society, both deliberately structured and spontaneously evolving, as they operate at a concrete local level. They encompass, among other structures, the world of work, the neighborhood, the mass media, agencies of government (local, state, and national), the distribution of goods and services, communication and transportation facilities, and informal social networks. (p. 515)
- A macrosystem refers to the overarching institutional patterns of the culture or subculture, such as the economic, social, educational, legal, and political systems, of which micro-, meso-, and exosystems are the concrete manifestations. Macrosystems are conceived and examined not only in structural terms but as carriers of information and ideology that, both explicitly and implicitly, endow meaning and motivation to particular agencies, social networks, roles, activities, and their interrelations. What place or priority children and those responsible for their care have in such macrosystems is of special importance in determining how a child and his or her caretakers are treated and interact with each other in different types of settings. (p. 515)

According to Bronfenbrenner (1977), an individual's development and behavior is a function of their exposure to these various settings. Events in one setting may influence the individual's behavior and development in another. For example, an experience in the classroom or in the informal peer group may change their pattern of activities and interactions with the family at home or have the reciprocal effect, which then leads to consequences for learning and development (Bronfenbrenner, 1977). In the same context, exposure to discrimination and prejudice in any of these settings may lead to implications for youth development.

Ajrouch and Awad (2019) drew on Bronfenbrenner's ecological model to highlight how factors in the microsystem and exosystem/macrosystem may either promote or protect against encounters of discrimination. The various levels of discrimination—individual, institutional/organizational, and cultural—experienced by youth may be applied to the ecological model (Ajrouch & Awad, 2019). Individual discrimination occurs when one person treats another differently because of the other individual's membership in a social group (Benokraitis & Feagin, 1995). Examples include the use of racial slurs, such as "camel jockey," "towel head," or "terrorist" (Ajrouch & Awad, 2019), and can also be evident in social exclusion (Awad & Amayreh, 2016). According to Ajrouch and Awad (2019), the individual level of prejudice encompasses the microsystem, including the relationships individuals have within their most immediate environment and involves family members and friends. This represents the very first point of socialization for children; children with origins different from mainstream America may learn about the possibility of unfair treatment from their families (Ajrouch & Awad, 2019). Depending on the family interaction, the family may serve as a negative source of self-image or as a source of a pride and positive identity (Ajrouch & Awad, 2019). In the case of Arab Americans, research shows a growing likelihood that youth are more likely to view themselves as distinct from white American than older Arab American individuals (Ajrouch & Jamal, 2007).

The second level is institutional/organizational discrimination (Ajrouch & Awad, 2019), which involves the practices and policies of institutions that have an unequal impact on specific individuals depending on their social group membership (Benokraitis & Feagin, 1995). An example of organizational discrimination includes the enforcement of policies that prohibit girls from wearing any head coverings in school (Ajrouch & Awad, 2019). Ajrouch and Awad (2019) noted that because Islam and Arab identity is often conflated, anti-Muslim prejudice is often related to anti-Arab prejudice. An example in this case is the opposition to allowing major Muslim holidays to appear on public school district calendars (Ajrouch & Awad, 2019). Institutional/organizational levels of discrimination are contained within the more distal environment of the exosystem and involves the context of schools, neighborhoods, and wider society (Ajrouch & Awad, 2019). These environments influence the experience of discrimination through school curriculum materials, neighborhood characteristics, and government policy (Ajrouch & Awad, 2019). For Arab American youth, developmental conflict may occur when family has provided socialization practices toward a positive identity but portrayals in the school context are negative, leading youth to question their family practices. Children living in more ethnically dense neighborhoods may experience less discrimination than those living in more diverse neighborhoods. Then, when they are outside of their enclave, their treatment may be different, which may come as a shock to them. Governmental policies, such as the USA PATRIOT ACT, that specifically targeted Arab/Middle Eastern Americans and led to an increase in negative stereotypes also resulted in more discrimination (Ajrouch & Awad, 2019). Researchers indicate that Arab American families with children immediately affected by these policies (i.e., members being detained) likely experienced trauma (Furman, Lamphear, & Epps, 2016).

The third level is cultural discrimination (Ajrouch & Awad, 2019), which occurs when one group has the power to define pertinent cultural values for members of all social groups (Jones, 1997). Examples of cultural discrimination include the conceptions that tall and thin women who have blond hair and blue eyes are the epitome of beauty or that parenting styles in the West fostering independence from infancy are valued over parenting styles that foster interdependence on family (Ajrouch & Awad, 2019). Cultural discrimination can also be found in the media. For example, the absence of positive images of Arabs in American media combined with the multitude of adversarial images demonstrate the bias in depictions of Arabs to the American public, which essentially allows the negative images to resonate (Ajrouch & Awad, 2019). The cultural level of discrimination encompasses the macrosystem—including laws, customs, political beliefs, and mass media—and emphasizes the significance of the larger systems level in youth development (Ajrouch & Awad, 2019). Ajrouch and Awad (2019) discussed how discrimination in the macrosystem environment can effect development as early as the womb. For example, Lauderdale (2006) found that women with Arabic names were the only participants to have an increased risk of low birth weight or preterm births in the 6 months following 9/11 compared to 6 months prior to the events. A culture of hostility was cultivated by negative stereotypes in the larger social setting, which led to stressors experienced by expectant mothers and had dire consequences on their child's development (Ajrouch & Awad, 2019).

Negative stereotypes in the media have also been found to have profound effects on young children (Ajrouch & Awad, 2019). For example, Brown, Ali, Stone, and Jewell (2017) found that negativity bias against Arab Muslims was most profound in 6- to 8-year-old children. Further, even children with little knowledge regarding Arab Muslims held the same level of cultural stereotypes as adults. Similar evidence of negativity bias against Arabs in youth was found even prior to 9/11 (Wray-Lake, Syvertsen, & Flanagan, 2008). The use of these stereotypes to include or exclude certain social groups becomes especially pronounced during adolescence (Killen, Lee-Kim, McGlothlin, Stangor, & Helwig, 2002) and, consequently, relates to prejudice and fosters obstacles to inter-group relations (Ajrouch & Awad, 2019). Overall, the lack of positive media representations of Arab Americans serves as a risk factor to youth development as they search for broader societal representations to emulate beyond the socialization practices within the family level (Ajrouch & Awad, 2019).

Youth Identity Development

Ajrouch, Hakim-Larson, and Fakih (2016) discussed the various theoretical frameworks related to youth identity development. The establishment of a stable identity is central to development in youth, which is accomplished through exploration of various roles and ideals leading to commitments in identity, such as gender, ethnicity, religion, and occupation (Erikson, 1968; Marcia, 1966). The exploration and commitment processes ultimately lead to what Erikson refers to as an achieved ego-identity (Erikson, 1968). Such an achievement requires individuals to synthesize their childhood identifications in a manner that allows them to establish a reciprocal relationship with society while maintaining a sense of continuity with their self (Marcia, 1966). Developing a healthy identity through the processes of exploration and commitment is essential to an individual's mental health (French, Seidman, Allen, & Aber, 2006).

When it comes to identity, Baker and Shryock (2009) described the Arab American crisis:

> Arabs are set apart from the hyphenated American populations by aspects of U.S. foreign policy that drive a sharp ideological wedge between Arab and American identities. Specifically, Arabs and Muslims living in the United States repeatedly face situations in which their countries of origin, or Arabs and Muslims generally, are cast as enemies of the United States and its allies in the Middle East. As a result, Arab American identity is seen, by Arabs and non-Arabs alike, as an identity in question, as an identity that must continually prove itself. As a practical condition of citizenship, Arab Americans are expected to assure their fellow nationals that they belong, that they are loyal, that they are not a threat to national security, and so on. (p. 14)

In this case, the reciprocity is broken, and there is a lack of continuity with the self, which may ultimately lead to a crisis in identity development for Arab American adolescents, especially in terms of ethnic identity. Further complicating ethnic identity development is the paradox that Arab Americans face in negotiating their "Arabness" with "Whiteness" infringed upon them through ethnic classification systems in the United States.

Ethnic Identity Development

Ethnic identity has been found to contribute to the overall adjustment of minority group adolescents (Phinney, 1989) and is an integral part of an individual's social identity (Sellers, Smith, Shelton, Rowley, & Chavous, 1998). Phinney (1989) outlined ethnic identity development in minority group adolescents. Research on children has focused on how they learn the label for their own group and the various characteristics of that label (Phinney, 1989). In adolescence, this focus shifts to understanding the significance of one's group membership (Phinney, 1989). Factors such as increased cognitive abilities, more interactions outside their own communities, and increased concern regarding appearance and social life influence adolescent understanding of group membership (Phinney, 1989). These factors then contribute to increased awareness of social issues that make ethnicity more salient for minority youth (Phinney, 1989).

Many of the models developed regarding ethnic identity are intended for adults, as researchers have differing views on when the process begins (French et al., 2006). For example, Phinney (1989) posited that ethnic identity development begins during adolescence, while Cross, Strauss, and Fhagen-Smith (1999) based their model on development in adulthood. French et al. (2006) defined adolescence as a critical period for identity changes to be examined, as abstract reasoning abilities increase along with the desire to explore multiple facets of their identity.

Cross (1978) developed a model, the Nigrescence model, that shows a progression in stages of identity in black college students during the civil rights era. The model includes five stages moving from self-hatred to self-love (French et al., 2006): pre-encounter, encounter, immersion-emersion, internalization, and internalization-commitment (Cross, 1971). The initial stage, called the pre-encounter, is characterized by negative perceptions of one's own group membership (Phinney & Chavira, 1992). In this stage, group members do not give race or their racial group membership much thought and their exploration is very low (French et al., 2006). The encounter stage occurs with a negative event that removes the individual from their original views and makes them more aware of their racial identity (French et al., 2006). This leads to the immersion-emersion stage where individuals decide to identify as "black" and begin exploring the meaning of being and immersing themselves in everything that is "black" (French et al., 2006). The group member then enters the internalization stage, in which they have gained confidence and pride in their black identity and hold a positive esteem toward their group (French et al., 2006). In the internalization-commitment stage, group members carry their confidence and commitment to their racial group and use it to shift societal views from negative to positive and eliminate racism in society (French et al., 2006). This stage is also considered an achieved identity (Phinney & Chavira, 1992).

Due to lack of research on ethnic identity development in adolescents, Phinney (1989) sought to inform on this issue utilizing the existing literature and applying it to adolescents. Phinney (1989) studied a model that incorporates the concepts of Erikson (1968), Tajfel (1978), Marcia (1966, 1980), and Cross (1978) with a sample of adolescents to explore the developmental process. As discussed above, Erikson (1968) developed a theory of ego identity development, which was then operationalized by Marcia (1966, 1980). Ego identity development consists of four stages: identity-diffusion, moratorium, foreclosure, and identity achievement (Erikson, 1968; Marcia, 1966). Identity achievement tends to involve an identity crisis, which leads to exploration and a clear commitment to the self (Marcia, 1980). Phinney (1989) derived and summarized the four stages of ethnic identity development and conducted a study to determine whether these stages apply to adolescents of various ethnic backgrounds. The author provided the following definitions (p. 38):

- Diffuse: Little or no exploration of one's ethnicity and no clear understanding of the issues.
- Foreclosed: Little or no exploration of ethnicity, but apparent clarity about one's own ethnicity. Feelings about one's ethnicity may be either positive or negative, depending on one's socialization experiences.
- Moratorium: Evidence of exploration, accompanied by some confusion about the meaning of one's own ethnicity.
- Achieved: Evidence of exploration, accompanies by a clear, secure understanding and acceptance of one's own ethnicity.

Phinney (1989) then examined the relationship of ethnic identity to measures of ego identity and adjustment. Ninety-one American-born tenth-grade students from two high schools in Los Angeles participated in the study, including 14 Asian American, 25 black, 25 Hispanic, and 27 white. Within the Asian American sample, participants included Japanese, Chinese, Korean, Vietnamese, and Filipino origins. Hispanic participants were of Mexican and Central American origin. Only American-born students were included to minimize confounding identity variables.

Participants were interviewed using 20 questions that focused on the topic of ethnicity. The questions measured the extent of exploration of ethnicity, the commitment to an ethnic identity, and attitudes about ethnicity. Phinney (1989) utilized four scales from the Bronstein-Cruz Child/Adolescent Self-Concept and Adjustment Scale (Bronstein et al., 1987), including Self-Evaluation, Social and Peer Relations, Family Relations, and Sense of Mastery. The author measured ego identity using a scale that was adapted for the study population from an inventory created by Rosenthal, Gurney, and Moore (1981).

Results revealed that three of the four stages were reliably assigned to 60 of the 64 minority group subjects. Diffusion and foreclosure could not reliably be distinguished; therefore, were combined as an initial stage of development in which there has been no search. More than half of this group were in this initial stage characterized by lack of exploration of ethnic identity. For this group, ethnic identity was not seemingly an identity issue (Phinney, 1989). Then, there was a moratorium stage that was evident and was characterized by an increasing awareness of the importance and need to understand ethnic identity. One-fourth of the subjects showed evidence of being involved in ethnic identity search and were considered to be in the moratorium stage of ethnic identity development. The third stage was an achieved ethnic identity, where one-fourth of the participants demonstrated an ethnic identity search that resulted in a confident sense of self as a minority group member indicating this achieved identity. Scores for ego identity increased as ethnic identity stages increased. A one-way analysis of variance (ANOVA) by stages showed a significant difference in ego identity scores. The same patterns were found for all adjustment scale scores: with an increase in ethnic identity stage, there was an increase in self-evaluation, sense of mastery, social and peer interactions, and family relations scores. Results of a one-way ANOVA by stages showed significant differences in scores in all areas. No differences were found among ethnic groups.

Most of the research on development of ethnic identity in adolescents has been cross-sectional (Phinney & Chavira, 1992). These studies have generally shown higher levels of ethnic identity stage by age (Phinney, 1989, 1992; Phinney & Tarver, 1988), but research investigating the progression across time is relatively lacking. Therefore, Phinney and Chavira (1992) conducted a longitudinal study utilizing the sample from Phinney (1989) that examined changes in ethnic identity after 3 years.

Eighteen subjects (five Asian Americans, five Blacks, and eight Hispanics) from the previous study (Phinney, 1989) participated in the follow-up longitudinal study (Phinney & Chavira, 1992). Similar to the initial study, interview questions were used to measure participants' level of exploration and commitment to their ethnic identity. Participants were assigned to one of the three stages based on the evidence of exploration and commitment. Instead of the Bronstein-Cruz Child/Adolescent Self-concept and Adjustment Scale (Bronstein et al., 1987), the authors used the Rosenberg Self-esteem Inventory (Rosenberg, 1986) to measure self-esteem. Phinney and Chavira (1992) reported that of the eight participants who were initially in the unexamined stage 3 years ago, one remained at that stage, two moved to moratorium, and five moved to achieved identity. Four participants were in the moratorium stage 3 years ago; of those, one regressed to the unexamined stage, and three progressed to an achieved identity. Of the six participants with an achieved identity 3 years ago, five remained in this stage and one regressed to the unexamined stage.

Results showed that ethnic identity stage was significantly correlated with self-esteem at both the time points. Self-esteem at both the time points was significantly correlated; however, the authors did not find any relations between ethnic identity stages. The authors found an interaction where ethnic identity stage predicted self-esteem 3 years later. Inversely, self-esteem predicted ethnic identity stage 3 years later. Phinney and Chavira (1992) suggested that these interaction effects may indicate that (1) high self-esteem promotes exploration of ethnic issues, and (2) a better understanding of one's ethnicity may promote positive feelings about oneself. On the other hand, as found by Crocker and Major (1989), low self-esteem may lead to higher inclinations for adolescents to internalize negative stereotypes and feel negative about their group membership.

Subsequently, French et al. (2006) conducted a longitudinal study with adolescents examining changes in ethnic identity among African American, Latino American, and European American. Two dimensions of ethnic identity were examined including group-esteem and exploration. Group esteem was defined as "how one feels about being a member of one's racial or ethnic group" (p. 4). Exploration was defined as "how much an individual tries to find out what it means to be a member of one's racial or ethnic group" (p. 4). The study focused on continuous changes in ethnic identity rather than stages in order to examine more subtle changes across three time points.

Participants were selected from elementary and junior high/intermediate schools with high proportions of the student population being eligible for reduced or free lunch. All students who were in the grade prior to the transition to either junior or senior high school were recruited. School context and transition were utilized as an encounter in the process of ethnic identity development, an event that would catalyze the exploration phase. Three time periods of data collection were defined: Time 1 was the pre-transition year (between March and early June 1988 or 1989), Time 2 was taken about 10–12 months after the transition year began (January through May 1989 or 1990), and Time 3 was post-transition taken a year later. The sample consisted of 420 adolescents (258 early adolescents; 162 middle adolescents) from African American, Latino American, and European American backgrounds. Thirty percent of early adolescents began as fifth graders, and 70% as sixth graders. Sixty-three percent of middle adolescents began as eighth graders, and 37% as ninth graders. The authors used an ethnic identity measure adapted from Phinney (1989), which measured the constructs of group-esteem and exploration. Early adolescents were examined apart from middle adolescents.

Results of the early adolescent sample showed a significant increase in group-esteem over time, with the greatest change occurring over the transition year to junior high school. No changes in exploration were evident. There was a significant difference in group-esteem patterns with African American and Latino American students being significantly different from European American students with a greater increase over time.

Results of the middle adolescent sample showed a significant increase in both group-esteem and exploration over time. Group-esteem rose over time; however, the greatest change occurred over the transition from junior to senior high school. The pattern for exploration, on the other hand, revealed a steady increase. There was only a marginal difference by ethnic group with African Americans and Latino Americans increasing slightly more than European Americans across the three time periods.

French et al. (2006) concluded that group-esteem and exploration followed different pathways with group-esteem rising for both early and middle adolescent samples and exploration rising only for middle adolescents. They speculated that the rising group-esteem levels in younger adolescents may not represent a movement toward achieved identity, as there was no evidence of exploration. Rather, this cohort's group-esteem was a result of the mere acceptance of family teachings regarding group membership. In addition, the high schools in this study were considered more ethnically diverse than the elementary and junior high schools. As such, the middle adolescent participants experienced a change in the ethnic composition of the school when they made the transition to high school. The authors considered this an encounter that heightened racial awareness and, therefore, served as a catalyst for the exploration process. Consequently, a rise was found in exploration for this cohort with subsequent rises in group-esteem the following years. Because the elementary and junior high schools were considered more ethnically homogenous, the same effect of racial awareness was not seemingly encountered. Research shows that students reported more instances of discrimination in schools with more diverse settings (Rosenberg, 1962) and that institutional racism in schools may become more evident with increasing student diversity (Fine, 1997). Such events may serve to stimulate an encounter and the exploration process (French et al., 2006).

Ethnic identity is a major developmental endeavor for ethnic minority youth (Mirpuri et al., 2019). The importance of studying ethnic identity development lies in evidence that the construct is related to various aspects of well-being. For example, Sheldon, Oliver, and Balaghi (2015) studied the relationship between ethnic identity and psychological well-being in Arab American emerging adults. The sample consisted of 174 Arab Americans between the ages of 18 and 29 years. The authors used the Multigroup Ethnic Identity Measure (Phinney, 1992) to assess various aspects of ethnic identity, including affirmation and belonging, other-group orientation, exploration, and commitment. The Ryff Scales of Psychological Well-Being (Ryff, 1989) measured well-being with the subscales of Self-Acceptance, Purposes in Life, and Personal Growth. Multiple regression analyses indicated that affirmation, belonging, and ethnic identity exploration were significant predictors of self-acceptance. Specifically, greater levels of affirmation and belonging led to greater self-acceptance; however, greater levels of exploration led to the lower levels of self-acceptance. Commitment was a significant predictor of purpose in life with stronger commitment levels associated with a greater purpose in life. Other group orientation significantly predicted personal growth with stronger levels of other group orientation showing stronger levels of personal growth. Results from this study were consistent with various ethnic identity theories that will be discussed shortly, which involve the relations of ethnic identity and well-being. Most areas of ethnic identity showed that increased levels correlated to increased levels of well-being with the exception of ethnic identity exploration and self-acceptance. The authors note that this finding was consistent with Erikson's and Phinney's theories of identity development in that exploration is a time of uncertainty and instability that individuals face through their journey of identity commitment. One important factor in this relationship between ethnic identity and well-being that was not investigated by Sheldon et al. (2015), and notably served as a limitation to their study, was the influences of discrimination.

Most of the research regarding Arab American youth has focused on development in relation to environmental factors, such as peer relationships, school environment, family relations, and discrimination (Britto, 2008). Britto (2008) discussed the multiple facets contributing to ethnic identity in Arab American youth. This includes religion, especially for Arab Muslim youth, and gender, where girls who wear the hijab—or head covering—have been found to feel the most vulnerable to discrimination and bullying (Britto, 2008). There are two reasons for religious affiliation differences in ethnic identity (Sheldon et al., 2015). First, Arab culture is highly embedded in Islam (Sheldon et al., 2015). Second, historical and present-day sociopolitical events have caused a divide between Christian and Muslim Arabs (Read, 2008). Therefore, it is critical for researchers to consider religious affiliation when studying ethnic identity in Arab American populations (Sheldon et al., 2015). For example, research has shown that Muslims are more likely to identify with their Arab heritage (Nassar-McMillan, Lambert, & Hakim-Larson, 2011), while Christians are more likely to identify as white rather than Arab (Read, 2003).

Research regarding ethnic identity formation in Arab American adolescents is lacking. However, one study provides some insight on this issue in a small sample of Arab American adolescents by demonstrating how gender may influence identity formation in this group (Ajrouch, 2004). Ajrouch (2004) conducted focus groups with ten Arab American adolescents in Dearborn, Michigan. The community of the students resided in was majority Arab, as was the school they attended. All participants were of the Muslim faith. Ajrouch (2004) held three focus groups over a 10-day period to investigate the formation of identity in these students.

The participants formed a continuum of identity with the terms "boater" and "white" at either extreme and placed themselves being somewhere in the middle. A "boater" was a person who was a recent immigrant to the United States and who was not yet familiar with the dominant culture. The term "white" was heavily tied with symbols of femininity. More specifically, discussions of "white" focused on the behavior of individual girls and the interactions between girls as well as between girls and boys. Furthermore, the author stated that the category suggests a racialized identity formed by the adolescents. The terms "boater" and "white" were used to describe what the adolescents had identified as the "others," those from who they have separated from themselves.

Results also indicated that the adolescents identified strongly with religion. The importance of religion was evident in defining appropriate behaviors for girls. Girls' behaviors were carefully scrutinized as to ensure they maintain honor, which was described as being central to herself, other family members, and the community (Ajrouch, 2004). In this sense, the girls essentially become the measure of "Arabness" (p. 383). Consequently, the female gender was also a strong factor in the identity formation of these adolescents.

Ajrouch (2004) maintained that a reason that girls were at the center of the definition of an American identity was the familial and community pressure on Arab American girls to avoid assimilation. The female participants discussed various behaviors that were tolerated by their family and community. They were also conflicted between expected and self-desired behaviors. They expressed the desire for acquiring autonomy, an American value that their male counterparts often enjoyed. Because the male participants in the group often had the choice of autonomy, the girls discussed the struggles of this double standard. The fact that the boys were able to behave the way they wanted and did not have to suffer the same consequences was completely unfair to the girl participants. Yet the boys believed that they were exempt from any of these restrictions due to religious reasons (Ajrouch, 2004). Here it is important to note that, because Arab culture and Islam are intertwined to a certain degree, religious and cultural reasons are often mistaken for each other, even within Arab communities. So, whereas one may perceive a reason as being religious, it really is more cultural and family dependent.

Ajrouch (2004) found that the Arab American adolescents in this study distinguished themselves from white Americans, regardless of them being labeled as white by the government. The Arab American girls in this study further distinguished themselves from white girls. This suggests that gender also has a major role in identity formation for Arab American adolescent girls. Ajrouch (2004) claimed that this finding is similar to findings with children of immigrants from Ireland, Poland, Italians, Asian Indians, Mexicans, and Filipinos, in that ethnic identity formation operates through gender relations, and girls often hold the role of cultural carriers, transmitters, and bearers of identity.

Various ethnic identity models exist and have been extensively studied with other ethnic minorities. Available ethnic identity models, however, have not been studied with Arab American adolescent populations (Britto, 2008). Therefore, it is unclear whether or not these models apply to them (Britto, 2008). Britto (2008) discussed the various types of ethnic identity models and reasons why they do not pertain to Arab American youth.

The first type of ethnic identity models focused primarily on the first-generation white ethnic groups who immigrated to the United States in 1920 and assimilated into the mainstream (Britto, 2008). Although Arab Americans are ethnically categorized as white by the government, they are persistently made aware of their "foreignness" (p. 855), which impedes their assimilation if that is their ultimate identity achievement. Therefore, these original models do not pertain to the experience of this population.

The next type of ethnic identity models focus on more recent immigrants of color, and the primary factor defining ethnicity is skin color (Britto, 2008). This model is not relevant for several reasons (Britto, 2008): Again, because of their categorization as white, Arabs are not technically immigrants of color. In addition, skin color is not a major determinant of Arab ethnicity.

The third type of models classify ethnic identity into four broad categories: national identity, American national identity, hyphenated American identity, and panethnic identity (Britto, 2008). Britto and Amer (2007) suggested that national identity and American national identity are national entities that do not apply to the category of Arab. Britto (2008) posited that the latter two categories—hyphenated American identity and panethnic identity—are minimally relatable. The hyphenated term "Arab-American" was developed as a result of political events in the 1960s and served to unite Arab immigrants and US-born Arabs under a shared heritage and history (Britto, 2008). Therefore, the term defines a bicultural identity that encompasses both American and Arab (Ajrouch, 2004), for which the American part cannot be ignored (Britto, 2008). A panethnic identity does address the ethnic identity factor for Arab Muslim youth; however, it does not cover the religious aspect, which is often a strong influence on the development of ethnic identity for this group (Britto, 2008). Therefore, for Arab Muslim youth, in particular, there are multiple dimensions of Arab Muslim identity that need to be addressed and consolidated in the development of an ethnic identity model, including an ethnic Arab dimension with strong cultural, historical, and social components as well as a religious component that is linked to ethnicity (Britto, 2008; Britto & Amer, 2007).

According to Erikson (1968), stigmatized minorities may internalize negative portrayals of the majority leading to the development of a negative identity. Tajfel (1978) suggested that stigmatized minorities may develop psychological conflict where they are faced with the choice of accepting these negative portrayals about their group or rejecting them and searching for their own identity. This leads to the discussion regarding the various theories on the relationship between identity and discrimination.

Social identity theory. Social identity consists of the aspects of an individual's self-image that derive from the social categories to which he perceives himself as belonging (Tajfel & Turner, 2001). Tajfel and Turner (2001) stated that the critical criteria for group membership are that the individuals define themselves and are defined by others as members of a group. The authors conceptualized a group as a collection of individuals who perceive themselves to be members of the same social category, share some emotional involvement in this common definition of themselves, and achieve some degree of social consensus about the evaluation of their group and of their membership of it (Tajfel & Turner, 2001). According to Tajfel and Turner (2001), members use these social groups to identify themselves in social terms. Further, these identifications are relational and comparative as they define the member as similar to or different from—and as better or worse than—members of other groups (Tajfel & Turner, 2001). The authors presented the concept of social identity with the following assumptions (p. 40):

1. Individuals strive to maintain or enhance their self-esteem: they strive for a positive self-concept.
2. Social groups or categories and the membership of them are associated with positive or negative value connotations. Hence, social identity may be positive or negative according to the evaluations (which tend to be socially consensual, either within or across groups) of those groups that contribute to an individual's social identity.
3. The evaluation of one's own group is determined with reference to specific other groups through social comparisons in terms of value-laden attributes and characteristics. Positively discrepant comparisons between in-group and out-group produce high prestige; negatively discrepant comparisons between in-group and out-group result in low prestige.

Based on the above assumptions, Tajfel and Turner (2001) derived the following theoretical principles comprising social identity theory (p. 40):

- Individuals strive to achieve or to maintain positive social identity.
- Positive social identity is based to a large extent on favorable comparisons that can be made between the in-group and some relevant out-groups: the in-group must be perceived as positively differentiated or distinct from the relevant out-groups.
- When social identity is unsatisfactory, individuals will strive either to leave their existing group and join some more positively distinct group and/or to make their existing group more positively distinct.

Based on these principles, Tajfel and Turner (2001) hypothesized that pressures to evaluate one's own group positively through in-group/out-group comparisons lead social groups to attempt to differentiate themselves from each other. The authors defined three variables that influence intergroup differentiation in concrete social situations. First, the individual must have internalized their group membership as a part of their self-concept. Second, there must be a social situation that allows for intergroup comparisons that enable the selection and evaluation of the relevant relational characteristics. Third, in-groups only compare themselves to relevant out-groups, not every existing out-group. Out-group comparability variables include similarity, proximity, and situational salience (Tajfel & Turner, 2001).

Rejection-identification model. Branscombe, Schmitt, and Harvey (1999) conceptualized the rejection-identification model. The authors theorized that willingness to make attributions to prejudice negatively impacts well-being and increases hostility toward the dominant group; however, the willingness to make attributions to prejudice increases identification with minority group which, then, increases psychological well-being (Branscombe et al., 1999). Therefore, attributions to prejudice directly negatively affect well-being and indirectly positively affect well-being by increasing minority group identification (Branscombe et al., 1999). The effects of making attributions are dependent on the pervasiveness of prejudice and expectancies of future encounters of prejudice, one instance of discrimination may be coped with entirely differently than multiple instances (Branscombe et al., 1999).

This model is based on various theoretical perspectives in social psychology that predict that experiences with discrimination damage self-esteem in those affected (Branscombe et al., 1999; Crocker & Major, 1989). The process begins with a recognition of prejudice as rejection from the dominant group. This rejection is internalized leading to lower self-esteem (Cooley, 1902; Mead, 1934). In terms of protecting self-esteem and well-being, the model utilizes Crocker and Major's (1989) proposal that key factors in coping with prejudice and maintaining positive self-esteem in devalued groups were attributing negative outcomes to prejudice, selective devaluing of certain performance dimensions, and using in-group rather than out-group comparisons for evaluating success (Branscombe et al., 1999). Branscombe et al. (1999) suggested that in a single case of discrimination, individuals are more likely to discount the incident to protect their self-esteem; however, with more reoccurring and stable incidents, self-esteem is more likely to be negatively affected.

Implications of Ethnic Identity on Outcomes of Discrimination

The importance of studying ethnic identity lies in the evidence the current literature shows on the moderating impact it has on the association between ethnic discrimination and adolescent outcomes, including academic indicators, externalizing behaviors, and mental health among ethnic minority youth (Mirpuri et al., 2019). However, a literature review by Mirpuri et al. (2019) on these outcomes indicated that there are mixed results across studies, either results being inconsistent regarding effects or that the strength of the effects are mixed. Nevertheless, among academic indicators, there is evidence of a moderating effect on grades (e.g., Chavous, Rivas-Drake, Smalls, Griffin, & Cogburn, 2008) and school engagement outcomes (Wong, Eccles, & Sameroff, 2003). Research on mental health indicators has shown a moderating effect on self-esteem (Romero & Roberts, 2003; Umaña-Taylor, Tynes, Toomey, Williams, & Mitchell, 2015), depressive symptoms (Umaña-Taylor & Updegraff, 2007), anxiety (Tynes, Umaña-Taylor, Rose, Lin, & Anderson, 2012), and stress (Sellers, Caldwell, Schmeelk-Cone, & Zimmerman, 2003). The research on externalizing behaviors—such as anger and aggression—is rather scarce, as only two were found in their review (Mirpuri et al., 2019), and the results were inconsistent. While Umaña-Taylor, Wong, Gonzales, and Dumka (2012) found that ethnic identity had a protective effect for males among Latinx adolescents, Lee, Lee, Hu, and Kim (2015) found that a stronger ethnic identity among adopted Korean American adolescents exacerbated the relationship between discrimination and externalizing behaviors.

Multi-Dimensional Self-Concept Development in Adolescence

Marsh (1990) provided a historical overview of theories of the self. Prior to the 1980s, the self was viewed as a single global construct, which ignored the notion that a person could have multiple perceptions of competencies in several areas. For example, a person might perceive himself/herself as a good athlete, but perceive himself/herself as not competent in school. Therefore, this person would have a positive athletic self-concept but a negative academic self-concept. Using a global self-concept impedes investigators from being able to measure these different constructs of the self. Consequently, several theorists (James, 1890; Shavelson, Hubner, & Stanton, 1976) argued that the self was a multidimensional construct and could not be thought of as one whole construct. However, there was not enough evidence at that time to support the idea of the self as a multidimensional construct. This was due in part to the inconsistent results obtained from studies conducted on self-concept prior to 1980. Empirical support was weak for self-concept in relation to age and sex, academic achievement, social support, self-attributions, and interventions. Although at the time, investigators were beginning to believe that self-concept was not as pertinent to the normative development of people as they thought. However, such inconsistent findings seem now to have been due to the fact that self-concept was being measured as a global construct and the instruments being used to measure self-concept were not appropriate (Marsh, 1990).

As a result of these inconsistencies, the 1980s sparked an era of research in the area of self-concept that focused on the provision of evidence to support the multidimensional self-concept. Researchers came to believe that self-concept cannot be understood fully without taking into consideration the multidimensionality of the self (Marsh, 1990). Shavelson et al. (1976) presented a multidimensional and hierarchical model developed from the review of existing research on self-concept and existing instrumentation. According to Shavelson et al. (1976), self-concept is a person's perceptions of him/herself, which are formed through experience with, and interpretations of, one's environment. Appraisals by significant others, reinforcements, and attributions for one's own behavior influence one's self-concept.

Shavelson et al. (1976) identified seven additional major factors that define their self-concept model:

1. It is organized or structured, in that people categorize the vast amount of information they have about themselves and relate these categories to one another.
2. It is multifaceted, and the particular facets reflect a self-referent category system adopted by a particular individual and/or shared by a group.
3. It is hierarchical, with perceptions of personal behavior at the base moving to inferences about self in subareas (e.g., English and mathematics components contribute to academic self-concept, whereas physical, social, emotional components contribute to nonacademic self-concept), and then to inferences about the self in general.
4. The hierarchical general self-concept, the apex of the model, is stable, but as one descends the hierarchy, self-concept increasingly becomes situation-specific and less stable.
5. Self-concept increasingly becomes multifaceted as the individual moves from infancy to adulthood.
6. Self-concept has both a descriptive and an evaluative aspect, such that individuals may describe themselves ("I am happy") and evaluate themselves ("I do well in mathematics").
7. Self-concept can be differentiated from other constructs such as academic achievement (Marsh, 1990; pp. 83–84).

The multidimensional, hierarchical self-concept is currently well received in the literature and has incurred significant empirical support (e.g., Bracken, Bunch, Keith, & Keith, 2000; Delugach, Bracken, Bracken, & Schicke, 1992; Jackson & Bracken, 1998). For example, Bracken et al. (2000) conducted a factor analysis on five established multidimensional self-concept instruments in attempt to restructure them into a proposed model of self-concept consisting of a global self-concept factor and six domain factors: physical, competence, affect, social, academic, and family. Five different self-concept scales were administered to 221 students. A factor analysis of the resulting 29 derived subscales indicated strong loadings on the global factor and the six dominant factors, which corresponded with the proposed theoretical model. The results from this study provide strong support for a multidimensional self-concept model across the instruments that were investigated.

The current understanding of self-concept is that it is indeed a multidimensional construct. Such a multidimensional focus allows researchers to develop a profile of self-evaluations across multiple domains for individuals or for particular groups of interest (Harter, 1999). This focus also allows researchers to examine whether the perceptions of some domains are more predictive of global self-concept than others.

Harter (1999) outlined the development of self-concept throughout the period of adolescence, including early, middle, and late adolescence. There is debate in the literature as to at what age adolescence begins (Ellis & Davis, 1982). Generally, the age range is between 13 and 18 years. However, researchers have not come to an agreement on exactly when adolescence starts because each child develops differently. For example, one child might reach puberty at 12 years while another might not reach that level until the age of 14 years. Therefore, the age ranges in this discussion are not specified because there is no set age range for the three stages of adolescence.

Researchers claim that during the early adolescent period, the self becomes increasingly differentiated with an abundance of selves that differ depending on the social situations, including the self with friends, classmates, teachers, siblings, parents as well as the self as a student, employee, athlete, and so on (Ellis & Davis, 1982; Rosenberg, 1986). This multidimensional self results in adolescents having differing—and at times conflicting—views of themselves within different social contexts. For example, adolescents may like themselves a lot with friends, but dislike themselves with parents. Such conflicting feelings could be due to perceiving positive support from friends but negative support from parents. In addition to having different feelings about themselves in different contexts, they are also likely to be treated differently by those in different social contexts. Consequently, "adolescents become very sensitive to the potentially different opinions and standards of the significant others in each context" (Harter, 1999, p. 67). The content of self-representations in early adolescents is focused on social skills that affect interactions with others or the adolescent's social appeal and interpersonal characteristics (Damon & Hart, 1988).

During the middle adolescent period, individuals become extremely consumed with what others think of them (Elkind, 1967). The self becomes further multiplied and differentiated within various social contexts. For example, the adolescent defines herself/himself differently with really close friends, with a general group of friends, as well as with family. This can further complicate the development for adolescents making it more confusing and challenging to decide who or what they are, especially if they receive potentially contradictory messages from others in their differentiated social context and become confused about which attributes to adopt (Harter, 1999). They begin to recognize that they have both positive and negative characteristics, which can lead to instability, confusion, and inaccuracies in their perceptions of their self (Higgins, 1991). Adolescents in this period begin to compare themselves with others in differential social contexts. For example, Buddin (1998) found that adolescents develop different levels of self-worth with their mothers and fathers in relation to the perceived feedback they received from each source. Furthermore, adolescents may attempt to change their behavior to seek approval from their social sources. For example, if an adolescent wanted to start doing her homework more often to please her parents, she may also be displeasing her friends by doing well in school despite pleasing her parents (Harter, 1999). This example illustrates the struggles of adolescents during this period trying to gain approval from two contradictory social contexts. They struggle to decide which one to adopt.

During the late adolescent period, contradictory characteristics described in the previous period are no longer seen as contradictory, as the adolescent accepts these differences as something that is normal (Harter, 1999). The inconsistencies in their differentiated selves become normalized. More specifically, adolescents find value in their inconsistent differentiated selves (Damon & Hart, 1988). They begin to realize that it is normal to be different in various roles with others. Adolescents' characteristics in this period begin to "reflect personal beliefs, values, and moral standards that have become internalized or, alternatively, constructed from their own experiences" (Harter, 1999, p. 79). Self-concept becomes more balanced with a stable view of both positive and negative attributes. Their selves are defined with more accuracy, and they are able to accept limitations of their self. Finally, with a futuristic outlook, these late adolescents begin to construct their own standards of self and follow their own aspirations.

Although there is a wealth of research on self-concept in various other ethnic minority groups, the research on the development of self-concept in Arab American students is very limited. Only two studies that investigated self-concept in Arab American students were found in the literature, and the results are conflicting. These studies were cross-sectional and did not investigate developmental changes over time. Al-Khatab (1999) conducted a study to explore the self-concept of a convenience sample of 237 Arab American adolescents (119 female) in grades 6 through 12. Students were from Detroit, Michigan, Lexington, Kentucky, and San Diego, California. Participants were asked to complete the Self-Perception Profile for Children (Harter, 1985) to measure self-concept in six domains: scholastic competence, social acceptance, athletic competence, physical appearance, and behavioral conduct.

According to Al-Khatab (1999), scores above 2.5 indicated a positive self-concept and scores below that indicated a low self-concept. This interpretation of Harter's scale differs from that of other researchers in that scores 3 and above were positive and scores below 3 were considered a negative self-concept (Kloomok & Cosden, 1994). Results indicated that the overall self-concept profile of these students was positive, suggesting that Arab American students perceive themselves positively. All responses were above 2.5 in all domains, indicating a positive self-concept according to the author's interpretation of the scores. Athletic competence and physical appearance scores were significantly higher for boys than girls, while behavioral conduct was significantly higher for girls. Social acceptance scores for sixth graders were significantly higher than all the other grades. Al-Khatab (1999) suggested that this finding is comparable to other findings in that self-concept decreases when children reach adolescence.

There are several limitations to this study that call for a cautious interpretation of the results. First, over half of the sample was from a city where there is a significant population of Arab Americans. In other words, these students are considered the majority in that location. Perhaps that sample of students had a positive profile due to a large population of Arab Americans in that city, resulting in higher tolerance in school. In schools where there is a large community of Arab Americans, such as Dearborn and Detroit, fewer incidents of discrimination are reported (Ibish, 2003). Such communities are better equipped to prevent anti-Arab incidents due to an established working relationship between Arab American leaders, school, police officials, and other community organizations (Ibish, 2003). Consequently, that sample of students' self-concept may be higher than students who have encountered such discrimination and prejudice. Additionally, this study examined self-concept alone, without investigating the relationship with external factors. Finally, this study was conducted before the events of 9/11; examining the self-concept in Arab youth after these events is necessary.

Kovach and Hillman (2002) examined self-esteem among other factors in Arab, African, and European American high school students. Self-concept and self-esteem are not interchangeable constructs; however, they are related. An individual with high self-concept might be expected to also hold high self-esteem, or low self-concept and low self-esteem. Kovach and Hillman (2002) found results that conflict with the results from the study conducted by Al-Khatab (1999). Participants completed the Rosenberg Self-esteem Scale (Rosenburg, 1965) to measure self-esteem. The authors found that Arab American students had the lowest self-esteem compared to the other two ethnic groups. They were also more likely to attribute negative feedback from out-group members to prejudice. Arab American students nominated prejudice as a causal explanation for negative outcomes or feedback more frequently than African American students. In addition, they frequently endorsed prejudice as a reason for failure like African American students, which was different from European American students. Girls had significantly higher scores for self-esteem than boys for all groups, unlike findings of Al-Khatab (1999). It should be noted that there was unequal sample sizes for the ethnic groups examined. The sample of African American students was much larger than the Arab and European American sample. Additionally, the Arab American sample was not representative of all the countries in the Arab world with the majority being from Iraq and Lebanon. This limits the generalizability of the results to various Arab populations. Finally, this study used samples from only three different schools, which also significantly reduces the generalizability of the findings. This study warrants replication with the use of a larger, more representative sample of youth from various Arab countries of origin.

As individuals progress through adolescence, they can become consumed with the opinions and expectations of others in various roles, such as parents, classmates, close friends, and teachers. Even more, the interrelationships and social interactions with others may lead to affective reactions to the self. Depending on the quality of the relationship, these interactions could potentially harm or improve the adolescent's self-concept. For example, the literature discusses several factors that, in accordance with the symbolic interaction theory, are related to the self-concept in adolescents. These factors—perceived social support and experiences of prejudice and discrimination—are outlined throughout the next section of this chapter.

The Symbolic Interaction Theory of Self-Concept

The symbolic interaction theory regards the self-concept as a social construction, conceived through social interactions or symbolic interactions with others (Baldwin, 1897; Cooley, 1902; Mead, 1925, 1934). According to this theory, an individual assumes the opinions that others are perceived to hold toward himself/herself. For example, if a child perceives that his mother feels that he is a good person, then the child will hold that opinion about himself. Likewise, if a child perceives that his teacher thinks he is not intelligent, then the child will hold that opinion about himself. Whereas Cooley (1902) theorized that significant others affect this process, Mead (1925) theorized that others in general could have the same effect. Research, which will be discussed later in this chapter, indicates that both significant others, such as parents and close friends, and general others, such as teachers and classmates, have an influence on self-concept (Demaray & Malecki, 2002, 2003; Forman, 1988).

The symbolic interaction theory has been supported empirically. Research has found that social interactions influence the self-concept, especially during the period of adolescence. Perhaps this is due to the dramatic developmental changes in adolescence that result from puberty, physical changes, cognitive development changes, and shifting social expectations (Harter, 1999). Evidence shows that adolescents report differing levels of self-concept across different relationships. Harter, Bresnick, Bouchey, and Whitesell (1997) examined perceptions of self-worth in high school students across four contexts: parents, teachers, male classmates, and female classmates. The authors obtained a clear, four-factor solution indicating that the adolescents made clear distinctions among their feelings of self-esteem in these relationships. The differentiated self-concept across relational contexts can be seen especially with youth from ethnic minority groups (Cooper, Jackson, Azmitia, Lopez, & Dunbar, 1995).

Cooper et al. (1995) discussed the challenges of minority groups having to move between multiple contexts, including members of their own ethnic group and members of the dominant culture. These challenges can be worse for some more than others, depending on the support from these social contexts. For youth who have teachers, peers, and families with congruent values, they can more easily move between their multiple contexts. When youth have social contexts with incongruent values, some develop a bicultural standpoint and adapt to the world of their ethnic group and the dominant group while others find the transition more difficult and sometimes impossible (Harter et al., 1997). Arab American adolescents might be expected to experience the same challenges.

Perceived social support. Perceived social support is defined as the perception of positive regard from others or the regard that others manifest toward the self. Beginning in the early 1900s, Cooley (1902) theorized that a person's self-concept is influenced by their social interactions with others. Since then, there has been a significant amount of literature and research supporting this relationship. Perceived social support from others has been found to be significantly related to students' self-concept. For this chapter, the discussion will be focused on a sample of the relevant literature regarding the perceived social support of teachers and peers in its relation with the self-concept. Students spend the majority of their day at school with their teachers and classmates, who provide an important source of interpersonal relationships. The teacher–student relationship can influence academic achievement and psychological factors. According to the symbolic interaction theory, the quality of this relationship can have a significant effect on the self-concept of students. For adolescents who are struggling with their differentiated selves and are trying to negotiate the changing relationships with parents and peers, teachers can mediate these struggles and act as a protection to the adolescent by providing support and guidance. This protection could potentially serve to improve the self-concept of adolescents. On the other hand, if no support is provided by the teacher, then this could serve to harm the self-concept.

The literature suggests that there is a significant relationship between perceived social support from different sources and self-concept (e.g., Demaray & Malecki, 2002; Demaray, Malecki, Rueger, Brown, & Summers, 2009; Reddy, Rhodes, & Mulhall, 2003). Research also provides evidence of a directional influence on self-concept according to perceived social support (e.g., Reddy et al., 2003). Specifically for adolescents, teachers and peers appear to have an overwhelming influence on the self-concept. Thus, it seems that the relationships and experiences students have at school, and how students perceive those relationships, can significantly impact how they perceive themselves.

An unsupportive environment with a lack of caring relationships where individuals have no one to relate to has proven to be a risk factor in adolescent development (Jessor, Van Den Bos, Vanderryn, Costa, & Turbin, 1995). The quality of support perceived may also be related to perceived discrimination from support systems in school; specifically, teachers and/or peers who treat an ethnic minority adolescent fairly may be perceived as more supportive, whereas those who treat the adolescent prejudicially may be viewed as unsupportive. Such discriminatory behaviors communicate that ethnic group members are different and do not belong to the majority, leading these individuals to believe that they are devalued because of their membership (Wong et al., 2003).

Experiences of discrimination. The stigma hypothesis states that the internalization of stigma, or minority status, leads to lower self-concept in minority groups (Twenge & Crocker, 2002). The status of being a minority becomes internalized with experiences of prejudice and discrimination. According to the stigma hypothesis, levels of self-concept in ethnic minority groups should correspond to the degree to which members of these groups are stereotyped or devalued by the majority or dominant group. The stigma hypothesis stems from the symbolic interaction theory in that self-concept develops from other people's perceptions of the self.

Research has shown that an individual's self-concept is closely linked to the devaluation of their ethnic minority groups (Twenge & Crocker, 2002). The relationship between self-concept and minority status—as well as discrimination—has been well-documented in the literature for African, Latino, and Asian Americans (e.g., Armenta & Hunt, 2009; Branscombe & Ellemers, 1998; Jasinskaja-Lahti, Liebkind, Jaakkola, & Reuter, 2006; Liebkind & Jasinskaja-Lahti, 2000). For example, Armenta and Hunt (2009) examined the effects of perceived personal and group discrimination on self-esteem in Latino(a) adolescents. To measure perceived personal discrimination, participants were asked to respond to the following statement: "I experience discrimination because of my ethnicity." A similar statement was used for group discrimination: "Other people of my ethnicity experience discrimination because of their ethnicity." Participants were asked to respond to these two items on a 6-point scale where a rating of 1 means the subject strongly disagrees and a rating of 6 means they strongly agree. Self-esteem was measured by the Rosenberg Self-Esteem Inventory (Rosenburg, 1965). Results indicated that subjects who perceived high perceptions of personal discrimination had low self-esteem, which is in line with symbolic interaction theory and the stigma hypothesis. However, high perceptions of group discrimination were related to higher self-esteem. The authors suggested that this was in line with the rejection-identification model, which states that discrimination of one's ethnic group leads them to identify more strongly with that group which, in turn, leads to higher self-esteem.

Developmental Consequences of Discrimination in Schools

Brenick, Schachner, Carvalheiro, and Karr (2019) identified consequences of developmental outcomes as a result of prejudice and discrimination in the schools. The authors noted that prejudice and discrimination have acute and long term consequences with implications for development through middle and high school and into adulthood. Brenick et al. (2019) cited psychological, social, physical, behavioral, and academic consequences of these experiences and discussed the existing research regarding these issues. The research presented does not explicitly include Arab American youth. The literature regarding discrimination and development outcomes has largely focused on other ethnic minority groups. The body of research focusing on Arab American adolescents is relatively scarce. It is important to understand the potential effects of discrimination, and therefore, we must look to the evidence available regarding other ethnic groups. Looking to the available research on other ethnic minority groups may aid in the understanding of potential processes, comparatively speaking, whether the evidence translates to the experiences of Arab American youth.

Research shows that experiencing discrimination in school is related to various factors of psychological maladjustment in youth, including—but not limited to—lower self-concept, higher depression, social anxiety, and loneliness (Brenick et al., 2019). For example, Wong et al. (2003) examined the relationship between racial discrimination at school and changes in academic and psychological functioning in a sample of African American adolescents. Data was recorded over two time periods, at the beginning of the seventh grade and at the completion of the eighth grade. Wong et al. (2003) found that discrimination at school from peers and teachers predicted academic self-concept, increases in depression and anger, and decreases in self-esteem and psychological resiliency. Experiences of discrimination were found to be potential risks to academic motivation, positive mental health, and self-esteem.

Niwa, Way, and Hughes (2014) conducted a longitudinal study with 585 Dominican, Chinese, and African American adolescents to investigate the relationship between perceived ethnic-racial discrimination and psychological adjustment. Discrimination was categorized by adults and by peers. Two clusters were found for adult discrimination. The first cluster involved a low-stable group with adolescents who did not perceive adult discrimination over time, while the second cluster involved a moderate-stable group with adolescents who perceived moderate, stable adult discrimination over time. The authors found significant differences between these two groups with the moderate-stable group perceiving significantly higher levels of discrimination by adults. Furthermore, boys were 1.6 times more likely than girls to be in the moderate-stable cluster. The authors speculate that the stability of adult discrimination profiles may be a result of social norms regarding explicit racist behavior; in other words, adults, especially in education, may be more likely to discriminate against adolescents implicitly (Niwa et al., 2014).

For peer discrimination, a three-group model was chosen (Niwa et al., 2014). The first cluster involved adolescents who perceived little to no peer discrimination, low-decreasing, with a decrease in perceptions through the 3 years. The second group, moderate-decreasing, represented moderate experiences with decreasing perceptions throughout the three time points. The third group, high-decreasing, involved high perceptions of peer discrimination at the initial stage of the study and a drop of perceptions by the end of the study. There were significant differences in perceptions of peer discrimination across groups. Boys were almost three times more likely to be in the moderate-decreasing group. Differences in ethnicity were found with Chinese Americans being 1.6 times more likely and Dominican Americans almost half as likely as African Americans to be in the high-decreasing cluster. Niwa et al. (2014) indicate that their results supported the literature regarding bullying and peer victimization that proposes a dramatic increase in events followed by a gradual decrease, especially for the high-decreasing cluster.

Niwa et al. (2014) reported, in terms of psychological adjustment, that adolescents in the moderate-stable adult discrimination group were more likely to have lower self-esteem and higher depressive symptoms than those with no experiences. Adolescents in the moderate- and high-decreasing peer discrimination groups were more likely to have lower self-esteem than those with no experiences. Only differences in depressive symptoms were found between moderate-decreasing and no peer discrimination groups with moderate-decreasing having significantly higher symptoms. No differences were found between high- and low-decreasing clusters. The authors suggest that this finding may imply that adolescents experiencing high levels of peer discrimination have become desensitized, lessening the effects of these experiences.

Another longitudinal study by Zeiders, Umaña-Taylor, and Derlan (2013) examined changes in self-esteem and depressive symptoms across the high school years among Latino adolescents. Data was accrued at four time points over a 4-year time period. The authors utilized the Rosenberg Self-Esteem Scale (Rosenberg, 1979) to measure self-esteem, the Center for Epidemiological Studies Depression Scale (Radloff, 1977) to assess depression symptoms, and a revised version of the Perceived Discrimination Scale (Whitbeck, Hoyt, McMorris, Chen, & Stubben, 2001) to measure the degree of perceived experienced ethnic discrimination.

Results indicated an increase in self-esteem over time and a decrease in depressive symptoms. Interrelations among self-esteem and depressive symptoms across time were high for both male and female adolescents. High levels of perceived ethnic discrimination were associated with lower self-esteem and higher depressive symptoms across each time point for male adolescents, but only related to higher depressive symptoms and time 2 and time 4 for female adolescents. Perceived ethnic discrimination significantly predicted self-esteem in male adolescents in early high school and changes in self-esteem growth for both male and female adolescents across the 4 years. Perceived ethnic discrimination also significantly predicted adolescents' depressive symptoms in early high school but did not predict changes in symptoms over time.

Benner and Graham (2013) examined antecedents and consequences of discrimination in Latino, African Americans, and Asian American adolescents. The authors found that racial and ethnic compositions of schools and neighborhoods influenced adolescents' perceptions of these racial and ethnic climates. For example, adolescents who viewed climates more negatively were more likely to perceive discriminatory treatment by school personnel, peers, and societal institutions. When it came to influential outcomes in development, each of these sources of discrimination was different. Greater discrimination from peers was associated with greater psychological maladjustment, including depressive symptoms, anxiety, loneliness, and global self-worth. Greater discrimination from school staff was associated with lower academic performance. Heightened racial awareness was only associated with societal discrimination, not school environment.

Research demonstrates that prejudice and discrimination in schools influence the social well-being of adolescents (Brenick et al., 2019), including the relationship quality with teachers and peers (Kiang, Witkow, & Thompson, 2016), which leads to lower social competence (Myrick & Martorell, 2011) and social isolation (Taylor & Peter, 2011). This can also lead to more severe feelings of being threatened by peers (Brenick et al., 2019). In the study by Niwa et al. (2014) discussed above, adolescents in the moderate-stable adult discrimination group were more likely to have lower best friendship quality, lower teacher–student relationship quality, and lower school belonging than those with no adult discrimination experience. Adolescence in the high-decreasing peer discrimination group were more likely to have lower teacher–student relationship quality and lower school belonging than those with no experience. The authors speculated that, because peer discrimination was common in middle school, the experiences may be normalized and have less influence on best friendship. However, since adult discrimination was less common, these experiences may have more impact on the amount of trust adolescents have to build close relationships in school, including close friends, teachers, and their school (Niwa et al., 2014).

Additionally, Wong et al. (2003) found that African American adolescents who experienced discrimination from their peers and teachers attributed more negative characteristics to their friends. Brenick et al. (2019) suggest that youth who are discriminated against can even be prevented from making social connections and, therefore, become socially isolated. For example, Tsai (2006) interviewed Taiwanese immigrant youth and found that their feelings of "otherness" and their chances of being discriminated against were increased by their school's English as a Second Language program.

Next, Brenick et al. (2019) identified the various physical consequences of school prejudice and discrimination. Physically, discrimination is associated with higher blood pressure and cortisol levels, which indicates higher levels of stress, which then leads to negative consequences for learning, memory, and risk for depression (Brenick et al., 2019). There is also evidence of associations with more somatic complaints such as headaches, stomach aches, and loss of appetite (Huynh & Fuligni, 2010). Research shows that these experiences do not need to be on a large scale basis, occur chronically, or even be overt in order for them to have physical effects (Brenick et al., 2019). For example, Huynh (2012) found that experiences with microaggressions were associated with increases in somatic symptoms in Latino and Asian American adolescents. Further, the more discrimination a student experiences, the worse their health condition may become (Brenick et al., 2019; Grollman, 2012).

In terms of behavioral consequences identified by Brenick et al. (2019), negative outcomes of discrimination in schools are problem behaviors and delinquency, including behaviors such as substance use, sexual activity, aggression, and skipping school. For example, Hershberger, Zapolski, and Aalsma (2016) found that higher levels of discrimination predicted higher levels of cigarette addiction, while Respress, Small, Francis, and Cordova (2013) found that black students were more likely to use marijuana when they perceived discrimination by their teachers. Further, an increase in sexual activity and substance use was associated with peer discrimination in Mexican American preadolescents (Sanchez, Whittaker, & Hamilton, 2016). Higher rates of delinquency were found in students who perceived that their student body at school was more prejudice (Le & Stockdale, 2011) and decreases in various forms of peer discrimination in high school were not found to be associated with any decreases in deviant behavior (Hughes, Del Toro, Harding, Way, & Rarick, 2016).

Ethnic differences in behavioral outcomes have also been found by researchers (Brenick et al., 2019). For example, Bogart et al. (2013) found that both black and Latino students had more problem behaviors associated with experiences of discrimination. Both black and Latino students endorsed more nonphysical aggression and retaliatory behavior than white students, while only black students reported more physical aggression. However, when accounting for discrimination experiences, the differences reduced significantly between black and white students. Furthermore, Latino students showed less behavior problems than white students. Brenick et al. (2019) indicated that such problem behaviors are likely to be interpreted as disruptive behaviors in school, leading to disparities in disciplinary action.

The final area identified and discussed by Brenick et al. (2019) was academic consequences. In addition to problem behaviors negatively impacting academic performance (Brenick et al., 2019), negative outcomes of prejudice and discrimination in school found in the literature include lower academic achievement, feeling disconnected to school, and decreased academic self-concept (Benner, Crosnoe, &

Eccles, 2015; Benner & Graham, 2013; Chavous et al., 2008; Wong et al., 2003). The academic outcomes discussed have not only been found in adolescents with direct discrimination experiences (Brenick et al., 2019); these consequences have been observed in bystanders who have either witnessed or just perceived discrimination in their school environment (Benner et al., 2015). Differential effects of discrimination have been found according to gender, socioeconomic status, and racial identity levels (Brenick et al., 2019).

For example, Chavous et al. (2008) examined the effects of classroom and peer discrimination in African American males and females longitudinally across two time points, eighth grade and eleventh grade. The authors examined males and females separately. Results indicated that, for boys, classroom discrimination in the eighth grade was negatively associated with GPA. Reported eighth grade discrimination predicted lower perceptions of school importance in the eleventh grade. Eleventh grade discrimination was also negatively associated with school importance in the same year. The relationship between classroom discrimination and school importance was significantly associated more negatively in males holding lower racial centrality, relative to higher racial centrality. The authors found a significant negative effect of classroom discrimination on academic self-concept in males with low socioeconomic status; however, the same association was not found in males of higher socioeconomic status.

In terms of peer discrimination for males, Chavous et al. (2008) found a negative association on GPA with the negative effects being more profound for boys with lower socioeconomic status and lower racial centrality. Peer discrimination was also a significant predictor of school importance with more profound negative effects in males with lower racial centrality. Finally, peer discrimination significantly predicted academic self-concept in male African American adolescents with the negative effect being stronger in males of low socioeconomic status. The authors rationalized these findings suggesting that earlier experiences of classroom discrimination were predictive of academic outcomes, whereas both earlier and later experiences of peer discrimination were related to these factors. A more profound risk of school discrimination was found among more disadvantage boys. Results were congruent with the literature on compensatory effects of racial centrality in relation to perceptions of school importance and academic self-concept, as well as the protective role centrality plays on the discrimination effects on male academic performance and school importance perceptions (Chavous et al., 2008).

Results from the African American female cohort were different from the males (Chavous et al., 2008). African American female students were found to have positive academic achievement in association with classroom discrimination in the eighth grade, but a negative association in the eleventh grade. Females reporting more classroom discrimination in the eleventh grade and having higher racial centrality also reported higher academic self-concept. With this result, the authors further found that for females with lower racial centrality, there was a positive association between classroom discrimination and academic self-concept; however, no relationship was found between these two factors in females with higher racial centrality.

In terms of peer discrimination for the female sample, experiences with peer discrimination were not associated with academic performance (Chavous et al., 2008). Peer discrimination was negatively related to school importance for females with higher socioeconomic status, but not those from low socioeconomic backgrounds. Experiences with peer discrimination also related to more negative perceptions of school importance in females of lower racial centrality, but not for those with higher centrality. Finally, peer discrimination across both the grades significantly predicted academic self-concept with the eighth-grade discrimination having a positive effect and eleventh grade having a negative effect. In conclusion, Chavous et al. (2008) indicated that more recent discrimination proved to have a more harmful effect for girls. Higher socioeconomic status was associated with greater vulnerabilities to discrimination effects on self-concept.

Conclusion

This chapter provided a thorough review of developmental processes in adolescents that are influenced by discrimination. The steps involved in each process were outlined, followed by dialogue that focused on the most relevant theoretical bases utilized in the research found on Arab American youth. Developmental processes have largely been studied with other ethnic minority groups. Research on developmental processes with Arab American youth are relatively lacking. This suggests that available developmental models may not be entirely relevant for these youth. Consequently, future research should examine these processes, specifically with Arab American youth, through longitudinal studies. With such research, relevant developmental models may be constructed and validated with these youth.

Theoretically, discrimination influences developmental factors, such as ethnic identity, self-concept, and general well-being. Theories differ, however, in the direction of influence. For example, while the rejection-identification model posits that ethnic minorities increase in ethnic identity with discrimination experiences and members seek refuge with their ethnic group, social identity theory posits that ethnic identity may decrease with experiences of discrimination, where ethnic minorities distance themselves from their ethnic group. Theories related to self-concept and general well-being largely suggest a damaging effect to these processes.

Indeed, the review of evidence shows that there is a relationship and influence of discrimination on development in ethnic minority groups. Even further, discrimination just within school systems has been found to have similar effects. The evidence available largely focuses on other ethnic minority groups. Studies on development in Arab American youth are severely lacking relative to other ethnic minority groups. Nevertheless, we must understand the potential effects of discrimination. The larger body of evidence available regarding other ethnic groups may be used to compare existing research on Arab youth to aid in the understanding of developmental processes and determine if the evidence potentially translates to their experiences. The evidence from other ethnic minority groups may also be used to inform future research studies focusing on Arab American youth in terms of methodology.

References

Ajrouch, K. J. (2004). Gender, race, and symbolic boundaries: Contested spaces of identity among Arab American adolescents. *Sociological Perspectives, 47*(4), 371–391.

Ajrouch, K. J., & Awad, G. H. (2019). An ecological approach to childhood prejudice: The case of Arab Americans. In H. E. Fitzgerald, D. J. Johnson, D. B. Qin, F. A. Villarruel, & J. Norder (Eds.), *Handbook of children and prejudice: Integrating research, practice, and policy* (pp. 147–159). Cham, Switzerland: Springer.

Ajrouch, K. J., Hakim-Larson, J., & Fakih, R. (2016). Youth development: An ecological approach to identity. In M. M. Amer & G. H. Awad (Eds.), *Handbook of Arab American psychology* (pp. 91–102). New York: Routledge.

Ajrouch, K. J., & Jamal, A. (2007). Assimilating to a white identity: The case of Arab Americans. *International Migration Review, 41*(4), 860–879. https://doi.org/10.1111/j.1747-7379.2007.00103.x.

Al-Khatab, A. (1999). In search of equity for Arab-American students in public schools of the United States. *Education, 120*, 254–266. Retrieved from http://proxy.lib.ohio-state.edu/login?url=http://search.ebscohost.com/login.aspx?direct=true&db=pbh&AN=2809113&site=ehost-live.

Armenta, B. E., & Hunt, J. S. (2009). Responding to societal devaluation: Effects of perceived personal and group discrimination on the ethnic group identification and personal self-esteem of Latino/Latina adolescents. *Group Processes & Intergroup Relations, 12*, 23–39. https://doi.org/10.1177/1368430208098775.

Awad, G. H., & Amayreh, W. M. (2016). Discrimination: Heightened prejudice post 9/11 and psychological outcomes. In M. M. Amer & G. H. Awad (Eds.), *Handbook of Arab American psychology* (pp. 63–75). New York: Routledge.

Baker, W., & Shryock, A. (2009). Citizenship and crisis. In DAAST (Ed.), *Citizenship and crisis: Arab Detroit after 9/11* (pp. 3–32). New York: Russell Sage Foundation.

Baldwin, J. M. (1897). *Social and ethical interpretations in mental development: A study in social psychology*. New York: Macmillan.

Benner, A. D., Crosnoe, R., & Eccles, J. S. (2015). Schools, peers, and prejudice in adolescence. *Journal of Research on Adolescence, 25*(1), 173–188. https://doi.org/10.1111/jora.12106.

Benner, A. D., & Graham, S. (2013). The antecedents and consequences of racial/ethnic discrimination during adolescence: Does the source of discrimination matter? *Developmental Psychology, 49*(8), 1602–1613. https://doi.org/10.1037/a0030557.

Benokraitis, N. V., & Feagin, J. R. (1995). *Modern sexism: Blatant, subtle, and covert discrimination* (2nd ed.). Englewood Cliffs, NJ: Prentice Hall.

Bogart, L. M., Elliott, M. N., Kanouse, D. E., Klein, D. J., Davies, S. L., Cuccaro, P. M., et al. (2013). Association between perceived discrimination and racial/ethnic disparities in problem behaviors among preadolescent youths. *American Journal of Public Health, 103*(6), 1074–1081. https://doi.org/10.2105/ajph.2012.301073.

Bracken, B. A., Bunch, S., Keith, T. Z., & Keith, P. B. (2000). Child and adolescent multidimensional self-concept: A five-instrument factor analysis. *Psychology in the Schools, 37*(6), 483–493.

Branscombe, N. R., & Ellemers, N. (1998). Coping with group-based discrimination: Individualistic versus group-level strategies. In J. K. Swim & C. Stangor (Eds.), *Prejudice: The target's perspective* (pp. 243–266). Boston, MA: Academic.

Branscombe, N. R., Schmitt, M. T., & Harvey, R. D. (1999). Perceiving pervasive discrimination among African Americans: Implications for group identification and well-being. *Journal of Personality and Social Psychology, 77*(1), 135–149. https://doi.org/10.1037/0022-3514.77.1.135.

Brenick, A., Schachner, M. K., Carvalheiro, D., & Karr, E. (2019). (no) space for prejudice! Varied forms of negative outgroup attitudes and ethnic discrimination and how they develop or can be prevented in the classroom. In H. E. Fitzgerald, D. J. Johnson, D. B. Qin, F. A. Villarruel, & J. Norder (Eds.), *Handbook of children and prejudice: Integrating research, practice, and policy* (pp. 315–330). Cham, Switzerland: Springer.

Britto, P. R. (2008). Who am I? Ethnic identity formation of Arab Muslim children in contemporary U.S. society. *Journal of American Academy of Child and Adolescent Psychiatry, 47*(8), 853–857.

Britto, P. R., & Amer, M. M. (2007). An exploration of cultural identity patterns and the family context among Arab Muslim young adults in America. *Applied Developmental Science, 11*(3), 137–150. https://doi.org/10.1080/10888690701454633.

Bronfenbrenner, U. (1977). Toward an experimental ecology of human development. *American Psychologist, 32*(7), 513–531. https://doi.org/10.1037/0003-066X.32.7.513.

Bronstein, P., Cruz, M., Cowles, C., D'Ari, A., Pienadz, J., Franco, O., et al. (1987). *A measure of child and adolescent self-concept and psychological adjustment.* Paper presented at the Annual Meeting of the American Psychological Association, New York.

Brown, C. S., Ali, H., Stone, E. A., & Jewell, J. A. (2017). U.S. children's stereotypes and prejudicial attitudes toward Arab Muslims. *Analyses of Social Issues and Public Policy, 17*(1), 60–83. https://doi.org/10.1111/asap.12129.

Buddin, B. (1998). *The effects of parental role modeling and support for voice on level of voice among high school students.* Doctoral dissertation, University of Denver, Denver, CO.

Chavous, T. M., Rivas-Drake, D., Smalls, C., Griffin, T., & Cogburn, C. (2008). Gender matters, too: The influences of school racial discrimination and racial identity on academic engagement outcomes among African American adolescents. *Developmental Psychology, 44*(3), 637–654. https://doi.org/10.1037/0012-1649.44.3.637.

Cooley, C. H. (1902). *Human nature and the social order.* New York: Charles Scribner's Sons.

Cooper, C. R., Jackson, J. F., Azmitia, M., Lopez, E., & Dunbar, N. (1995). Bridging students' multiple worlds: African American and Latino youth in academic outreach programs. In R. F. Macias & R. G. Garcia-Ramos (Eds.), *Changing schools for changing students: An anthology of research on language minorities* (pp. 211–234). Santa Barbara, CA: University of California Linguistic Minority Research Institute.

Crocker, J., & Major, B. (1989). Social stigma and self-esteem: The self-protective properties of stigma. *Psychological Review, 96*, 608–630.

Cross, W. E. (1971). Negro to Black conversion experience. *Black World, 20*, 13–27.

Cross, W. E. (1978). The Thomas and Cross models of psychological nigrescence: A review. *Journal of Black Psychology, 5*, 13–31. https://doi.org/10.1177/009579847800500102.

Cross, W. E., Strauss, L., & Fhagen-Smith, P. (1999). African American identity development across the life span: Educational implications. In *Racial and ethnic identity in school practices: Aspects of human development* (pp. 29–47). Mahwah, NJ: Lawrence Erlbaum Associates.

Damon, W., & Hart, D. (1988). *Self-understanding in childhood and adolescence.* New York: Cambridge University Press.

Delugach, R. R., Bracken, B. A., Bracken, M. J., & Schicke, M. C. (1992). Self concept: Multidimensional construct exploration. *Psychology in the Schools, 29*(3), 213–223.

Demaray, M. K., & Malecki, C. K. (2002). Critical levels of perceived social support associated with student adjustment. *School Psychology Quarterly, 17*, 213–241. https://doi.org/10.1521/scpq.17.3.213.20883.

Demaray, M. K., & Malecki, C. K. (2003). Importance ratings of socially supportive behaviors by children and adolescents. *School Psychology Review, 32*, 108–131. https://doi.org/10.1007/s10964-007-9258-3.

Demaray, M. K., Malecki, C. K., Rueger, S. Y., Brown, S. E., & Summers, K. H. (2009). The role of youth's ratings of the importance of socially supportive behaviors in the relationship between social support and self-concept. *Journal of Youth and Adolescence, 38*(1), 13–28.

Elkind, D. (1967). Egocentrism in adolescence. *Child Development, 38*, 1025–1034.

Ellis, D. W., & Davis, L. T. (1982). The development of self-concept boundaries across the adolescent years. *Adolescence, 17*, 695–710. Retrieved from http://search.proquest.com/docview/1295889693?accountid=9783.

Erikson, E. H. (Ed.). (1968). *Identity, youth, and crisis* (1st ed.). New York: Norton.

Fine, M. (1997). Witnessing whiteness. In M. Fine, L. Weis, L. C. Powell, & L. M. Wong (Eds.), *Off white: Readings on race, power and society* (pp. 57–65). Florence, KY: Taylor and Francis/Routledge.

Forman, E. A. (1988). The effects of social support and school placement on the self-concept of LD students. *Learning Disability Quarterly, 11*, 115–124. https://doi.org/10.2307/1510989.

French, S., Seidman, E., Allen, L., & Aber, J. (2006). The development of ethnic identity during adolescence. *Developmental Psychology, 42*(1), 1–10.

Furman, R., Lamphear, G., & Epps, D. (2016). *The immigrant other: Lived experiences in a transnational world*. New York: Columbia University Press.

Grollman, E. A. (2012). Multiple forms of perceived discrimination and health among adolescents and young adults. *Journal of Health and Social Behavior, 53*(2), 199–214. https://doi.org/10.1177/0022146512444289.

Harter, S. (1985). *Manual for the Self-Perception Profile for Children*. Denver, CO: University of Denver.

Harter, S. (1999). *The construction of the self: A developmental perspective*. New York: Guilford Press.

Harter, S., Bresnick, S., Bouchey, H. A., & Whitesell, N. R. (1997). The development of multiple role-related selves during adolescence. *Development and Psychopathology, 9*, 835–853. Retrieved from http://journals.cambridge.org/action/displayAbstract?fromPage=online&aid=43509&fulltextType=RA&fileId=S0954579497001466.

Hershberger, A., Zapolski, T., & Aalsma, M. C. (2016). Social support as a buffer between discrimination and cigarette use in juvenile offenders. *Addictive Behaviors, 59*, 7–11. https://doi.org/10.1016/j.addbeh.2016.03.003.

Higgins, E. T. (1991). Development of self-regulatory and self-evaluative processes: Costs, benefits, and tradeoffs. In M. R. Gunnar & L. A. Sroufe (Eds.), *Self-processes and development: The Minnesota Symposia on child development* (Vol. 23, pp. 125–166). Hillsdale, NJ: Erlbaum.

Hughes, D., Del Toro, J., Harding, J. F., Way, N., & Rarick, J. R. (2016). Trajectories of discrimination across adolescence: Associations with academic, psychological, and behavioral outcomes. *Child Development, 87*(5), 1337–1351. https://doi.org/10.1111/cdev.12591.

Huynh, V. W. (2012). Ethnic microaggressions and the depressive and somatic symptoms of Latino and Asian American adolescents. *Journal of Youth and Adolescence, 41*(7), 831–846. https://doi.org/10.1007/s10964-012-9756-9.

Huynh, V. W., & Fuligni, A. J. (2010). Discrimination hurts: The academic, psychological, and physical well-being of adolescents. *Journal of Research on Adolescence, 20*(4), 916–941. https://doi.org/10.1111/j.1532-7795.2010.00670.x.

Ibish, H. E. (2003). *Report on hate crimes and discrimination against Arab Americans: The post-September 11 Backlash September 11, 2001 - October 11, 2002*. Washington, D.C.: American Arab Anti-Discrimination Committee Research Institute.

Jackson, L. D., & Bracken, B. A. (1998). Relationship between students' social status and global and domain-specific self-concepts. *Journal of School Psychology, 36*(2), 233–246.

James, W. (1890). *The principles of psychology*. Chicago, IL: Encyclopedia Britannica.

Jasinskaja-Lahti, I., Liebkind, K., Jaakkola, M., & Reuter, A. (2006). Perceived discrimination, social support networks, and psychological well-being among three immigrant groups. *Journal of Cross-Cultural Psychology, 37*, 293–311. https://doi.org/10.1177/0022022106286925.

Jessor, R., Van Den Bos, J., Vanderryn, J., Costa, F. M., & Turbin, M. S. (1995). Protective factors in adolescent problem behavior: Moderator effects and developmental change. *Developmental Psychology, 31*(6), 923–933. https://doi.org/10.1037/0012-1649.31.6.923.

Jones, J. M. (1997). *Prejudice and racism* (2nd ed.). New York: McGraw-Hill.

Kiang, L., Witkow, M. R., & Thompson, T. L. (2016). Model minority stereotyping, perceived discrimination, and adjustment among adolescents from Asian American backgrounds. *Journal of Youth and Adolescence, 45*(7), 1366–1379. https://doi.org/10.1007/s10964-015-0336-7.

Killen, M., Lee-Kim, J., McGlothlin, H., Stangor, C., & Helwig, C. C. (2002). How children and adolescents evaluate gender and racial exclusion. *Monographs of the Society for Research in Child Development, 67*(4), i-129.

Kloomok, S., & Cosden, M. (1994). Self-concept in children with learning disabilities: The relationship between global self-concept, academic "discounting," nonacademic self-concept, and perceived social support. *Learning Disability Quarterly, 17,* 140–153. https://doi.org/10.2307/1511183.

Kovach, B. S., & Hillman, S. B. (2002, August 22-25). African and Arab American achievement motivation: Effects of minority membership. Paper presented at the 110th Annual Conference of the American Psychological Association, Chicago, IL.

Lauderdale, D. S. (2006). Birth outcomes for Arabic-named women in California before and after September 11. *Demography, 43*(1), 185–201. https://doi.org/10.1353/dem.2006.0008.

Le, T. N., & Stockdale, G. (2011). The influence of school demographic factors and perceived student discrimination on delinquency trajectory in adolescence. *Journal of Adolescent Health, 49*(4), 407–413. https://doi.org/10.1016/j.jadohealth.2011.02.003.

Lee, J. P., Lee, R. M., Hu, A. W., & Kim, O. M. (2015). Ethnic identity as a moderator against discrimination for transracially and transnationally adopted Korean American adolescents. *Asian American Journal of Psychology, 6*(2), 154–163. https://doi.org/10.1037/a0038360.

Liebkind, K., & Jasinskaja-Lahti, I. (2000). The influence of experiences of discrimination on psychological stress: A comparison of seven immigrant groups. *Journal of Community & Applied Social Psychology, 10,* 1–16. https://doi.org/10.1002/(SICI)1099-1298(200001/02)10:1<1::AID-CASP521>3.0.CO;2-5.

Marcia, J. E. (1966). Development and validation of ego-identity status. *Journal of Personality and Social Psychology, 3*(5), 551–558. https://doi.org/10.1037/h0023281.

Marcia, J. E. (1980). Identity in adolescence. In J. Adelson (Ed.), *Handbook of adolescent psychology*. New York: Wiley.

Marsh, H. W. (1990). A multidimensional, hierarchical model of self-concept: Theoretical and empirical justification. *Educational Psychology Review,* 2(2), 77–172.

Mead, G. H. (1925). The genesis of the self and social control. *International Journal of Ethics, 35,* 251–273.

Mead, G. H. (1934). *Mind, self, and society from the standpoint of a social behaviorist.* Chicago, IL: University of Chicago Press.

Mirpuri, S., Ray, C., Hassan, A., Aladin, M., Wang, Y., & Yip, T. (2019). Ethnic/racial identity as a moderator of the relationship between discrimination and adolescent outcomes. In H. E. Fitzgerald, D. J. Johnson, D. B. Qin, F. A. Villarruel, & J. Norder (Eds.), *Handbook of children and prejudice: Integrating research, practice, and policy* (pp. 477–499). Cham, Switzerland: Springer.

Myrick, S. E., & Martorell, G. A. (2011). Sticks and stones may break my bones: Protective factors for the effects of perceived discrimination on social competence in adolescence. *Personal Relationships, 18*(3), 487–501. https://doi.org/10.1111/j.1475-6811.2010.01320.x.

Nassar-McMillan, S. C., Lambert, R. G., & Hakim-Larson, J. (2011). Discrimination history, backlash fear, and ethnic identity among Arab Americans: Post-9/11 snapshots. *Journal of Multicultural Counseling and Development, 39,* 38–47. https://doi.org/10.1002/j.2161-1912.2011.tb00138.x.

Niwa, E. Y., Way, N., & Hughes, D. L. (2014). Trajectories of ethnic-racial discrimination among ethnically diverse early adolescents: Associations with psychological and social adjustment. *Child Development, 85*(6), 2339–2354. https://doi.org/10.1111/cdev.12310.

Phinney, J. S. (1989). Stages of ethnic identity development in minority group adolescents. *Journal of Early Adolescence, 9*, 34–49. https://doi.org/10.1177/0272431689091004.

Phinney, J. S. (1992). The multigroup ethnic identity measure: A new sclae for use with diverse groups. *Journal of Adolescent Research, 7*, 156–176.

Phinney, J. S., & Chavira, V. (1992). Ethnic identity and self-esteem: An exploratory longitudinal study. *Journal of Adolescence, 15*(3), 271–281. https://doi.org/10.1016/0140-1971(92)90030-9.

Phinney, J. S., & Tarver, S. (1988). Ethnic identity search and commitment in Black and White eighth graders. *The Journal of Early Adolescence, 8*(3), 265–277. https://doi.org/10.1177/0272431688083004.

Radloff, L. S. (1977). The CES-D scale: A self-report depression scale for research in the general population. *Applied Psychological Measurement, 1*(3), 385–401. https://doi.org/10.1177/014662167700100306.

Read, J. G. (2003). The sources of gender role attitudes among Christian and Muslim Arab-American women. *Sociology of Religion, 64*(2), 207–222. https://doi.org/10.2307/3712371.

Read, J. G. (2008). Discrimination and identity formation in post 9/11 era: A comparison of Muslim and Christian Arab Americans. In A. Jamal & N. Naber (Eds.), *Race and Arab Americans before and after 9/11: From invisible citizens to visible subjects* (pp. 305–317). Syracuse, NY: Syracuse University Press.

Reddy, R., Rhodes, J., & Mulhall, P. (2003). The influence of teacher support on student adjustment in the middle school years: A latent growth curve study. *Development and Psychopathology, 15*, 119–138. https://doi.org/10.1017/S0954579403000075.

Respress, B. N., Small, E., Francis, S. A., & Cordova, D. (2013). The role of perceived peer prejudice and teacher discrimination on adolescent substance use: A social determinants approach. *Journal of Ethnicity in Substance Abuse, 12*(4), 279–299. https://doi.org/10.1080/15332640.2013.836728.

Romero, A. J., & Roberts, R. E. (2003). The impact of multiple dimensions of ethnic identity on discrimination and adolescents' self-esteem. *Journal of Applied Social Psychology, 33*(11), 2288–2305. https://doi.org/10.1111/j.1559-1816.2003.tb01885.x.

Rosenberg, M. (1962). The dissonant religious context and emotional disturbance. *American Journal of Sociology, 68*(1), 1–10. https://doi.org/10.1086/223261.

Rosenberg, M. (1979). *Conceiving the self.* New York: Basic Books.

Rosenberg, M. (1986). *Conceiving the self.* Melbourne, FL: Krieger.

Rosenburg, M. (1965). *Society and the adolescent self-image.* Princeton, NJ: Princeton University Press.

Rosenthal, D. A., Gurney, R. M., & Moore, S. M. (1981). From trust on intimacy: A new inventory for examining Erikson's stages of psychosocial development. *Journal of Youth and Adolescence, 10*(6), 525–537. https://doi.org/10.1007/bf02087944.

Ryff, C. D. (1989). Happiness is everything, or is it? Explorations on the meaning of psychological well-being. *Journal of Personality and Social Psychology, 57*(6), 1069–1081. https://doi.org/10.1037/0022-3514.57.6.1069.

Sanchez, D., Whittaker, T. A., & Hamilton, E. (2016). Perceived discrimination, peer influence and sexual behaviors in Mexican American preadolescents. *Journal of Youth and Adolescence, 45*(5), 928–944. https://doi.org/10.1007/s10964-016-0420-7.

Sellers, R. M., Caldwell, C. H., Schmeelk-Cone, K. H., & Zimmerman, M. A. (2003). Racial identity, racial discrimination, perceived stress, and psychological distress among African American young adults. *Journal of Health and Social Behavior, 44*(3), 302–317. https://doi.org/10.2307/1519781.

Sellers, R. M., Smith, M. A., Shelton, J. N., Rowley, S. A. J., & Chavous, T. M. (1998). Multidimensional model of racial identity: A reconceptualization of African American racial

identity. *Personality and Social Psychology Review, 2*(1), 18–39. https://doi.org/10.1207/s15327957pspr0201_2.
Shavelson, R. J., Hubner, J. J., & Stanton, G. C. (1976). Self-concept: Validation of construct interpretations. *Review of Education Research, 46*, 407–441. https://doi.org/10.3102/00346543046003407.
Sheldon, J. P., Oliver, D. G., & Balaghi, D. (2015). Arab American emerging adults' ethnic identity and its relation to psychological well-being. *Emerging Adulthood, 3*(5), 340–352. https://doi.org/10.1177/2167696815597601.
Tajfel, H. (1978). *The social psychology of minorities*. New York: Minority Rights Group.
Tajfel, H., & Turner, J. (2001). An integrative theory of intergroup conflict. In M. A. Hogg & D. Abrams (Eds.), *Key readings in social psychology. Intergroup relations: Essential readings* (pp. 94–109). New York: Psychology Press.
Taylor, C., & Peter, T. (2011). "We are not aliens, we're people, and we have rights." Canadian human rights discourse and high school climate for LGBTQ students. *Canadian Review of Sociology, 48*(3), 275–312. https://doi.org/10.1111/j.1755-618x.2011.01266.x.
Tsai, J. H. (2006). Xenophobia, ethnic community, and immigrant youths' friendship network formation. *Adolescence, 41*(162), 285–298.
Twenge, J., & Crocker, J. (2002). Race and self-esteem: Meta-analyses comparing Whites, Blacks, Hispanics, Asians, and American Indians and comment on Gray-Little and Hafdahl (2000). *Psychological Bulletin, 128*, 371–408. https://doi.org/10.1037/0033-2909.128.3.371.
Tynes, B. M., Umaña-Taylor, A. J., Rose, C. A., Lin, J., & Anderson, C. J. (2012). Online racial discrimination and the protective function of ethnic identity and self-esteem for African American adolescents. *Developmental Psychology, 48*(2), 343–355. https://doi.org/10.1037/a0027032.
Umaña-Taylor, A. J., Tynes, B. M., Toomey, R. B., Williams, D. R., & Mitchell, K. J. (2015). Latino adolescents' perceived discrimination in online and offline settings: An examination of cultural risk and protective factors. *Developmental Psychology, 51*(1), 87–100. https://doi.org/10.1037/a0038432.
Umaña-Taylor, A. J., & Updegraff, K. A. (2007). Latino adolescents' mental health: Exploring the interrelations among discrimination, ethnic identity, cultural orientation, self-esteem, and depressive symptoms. *Journal of Adolescence, 30*(4), 549–567. https://doi.org/10.1016/j.adolescence.2006.08.002.
Umaña-Taylor, A. J., Wong, J. J., Gonzales, N. A., & Dumka, L. E. (2012). Ethnic identity and gender as moderators of the association between discrimination and academic adjustment among Mexican-origin adolescents. *Journal of Adolescence, 35*(4), 773–786. https://doi.org/10.1016/j.adolescence.2011.11.003.
Whitbeck, L. B., Hoyt, D. R., McMorris, B. J., Chen, X., & Stubben, J. D. (2001). Perceived discrimination and early substance abuse among American Indian children. *Journal of Health and Social Behavior, 42*(4), 405–424.
Wong, C. A., Eccles, J. S., & Sameroff, A. (2003). The influence of ethnic discrimination and ethnic identification on African American adolescents' school and socioemotional adjustment. *Journal of Personality, 71*(6), 1197–1232. https://doi.org/10.1111/1467-6494.7106012.
Wray-Lake, L., Syvertsen, A. K., & Flanagan, C. A. (2008). Contested citizenship and social exclusion: Adolescent Arab American immigrants' views of the social contract. *Applied Developmental Science, 12*, 84–92. https://doi.org/10.1080/10888690801997085.
Zeiders, K. H., Umaña-Taylor, A. J., & Derlan, C. L. (2013). Trajectories of depressive symptoms and self-esteem in Latino youths: Examining the role of gender and perceived discrimination. *Developmental Psychology, 49*(5), 951–963. https://doi.org/10.1037/a0028866.

Discrimination and Developmental Processes in Arab American Youth

Introduction

Arab American youth are one of the largest growing ethnic groups in the American school system. History shows that Arabs in America have long-faced discrimination, prejudice, and stereotyping, especially after the 9/11 terrorist attacks. Cultural stereotypes, misconceptions, and discrimination began with the immigration of this ethnic group to the United States and have become deeply rooted in American society, including the education system. The impact of these experiences on Arabs in America is likely to have dire consequences, especially for Arab youth as they begin to develop their identities and well-being. Therefore, the purpose of this chapter is to conduct a narrative review of the literature regarding the relations of discrimination and various aspects of development in adolescents of Arab descent in America. The chapter begins with a brief overview of Arab youth and their discrimination experiences. Then, a review of the research regarding this group is presented. Available studies on Arab youth have explored developmental processes of ethnic identity, self-concept, and general well-being in relation to discrimination. The research found on this group was relatively scarce but has been growing recently, which researchers suggest is a result of the backlash from mainstream society following 9/11. The review discusses the research found regarding experiences of discrimination throughout various settings including community and school in order to provide a broader perspective of their experiences.

An Overview of Arab Youth and Discrimination in America

The historical standard of misrepresentation of Arab cultures in America leads researchers to suggest that there is an expected risk to developmental processes in adolescents of Arab descent within multicultural society (Al-Hazza & Bucher,

R. Tabbah, *Arab American Youth*, Advancing Responsible Adolescent Development, https://doi.org/10.1007/978-3-030-66804-4_7

2010). There is evidence that negative perceptions and stereotypes in mainstream US media have led to a hostile environment and various forms of discrimination for Arabs in America (Bayoumi, 2009). Incidents of hate against Arabs in America did occur prior to 9/11, but rather infrequently; however, following the attacks, the number of incidents surged (Ibish, 2001). The latest report from the American Arab Anti-Discrimination Committee (ADC, 2011) stated a recent string of suicide deaths as a result of acts of discrimination and bullying in the K-12 system.

Negative perceptions have also been validated in empirical research. For example, Wray-Lake, Syvertsen, and Flanagan (2008) used open-ended questionnaires to collect data on sensitivity to images as enemies of America, experiences of prejudice and discrimination, and times when adolescent participants felt American. Results indicated that regardless of ethnic background, Arabs were nominated as enemies of America more than any other category. Over 69% of the Arab sample believed that Arabs in general or a specific Arab group were portrayed as enemies of America. Furthermore, out of the 93 Arab participants, 63 reported experiencing prejudice, where almost half were related to "being physically or outwardly identified as Arab" (p. 89). Consequently, adolescents of Arab descent in America are expectedly forming their identities in an environment surrounded by racism and prejudice with a keen awareness of the publics' low regard for the Arab American community (Read, 2008). Another study was conducted in Canada where Arab youth have strikingly similar experiences to those living in America (Finn, Hennebry, & Momani, 2018). Finn et al. (2018) investigated the lengths that Canadian Arab youth had to endure to minimize their visibility as a minority group, especially while traveling. More specifically, they examined the effects that heightened security precautions and the impact that racialization and securitization of Arabness had on Canadian Arab youths' thinking and behavior while traveling (Finn et al., 2018). The authors found three themes that emerged from the interviews with these youth. First, the youth utilized cultural dissociation to navigate racialization while traveling. For example, they differentiated markers of whiteness and Canadian secularism from markers of traditional and modern Arab culture and/or religion. Some expressed these differentiations as skin color; some with white skin tone were able to blend in with a white crowd, and others with darker skin tones were not afforded that privilege. The latter felt the need to differentiate by the way they dress and act (i.e., wearing baseball caps and hoodies). Another differentiating factor found was names. The participants were extremely conscious of how their names might be perceived while traveling. For example, one youth reported: "I try to say my family members' names as 'white' as possible…For example, Sara can be pronounced in an Arab or White way" (p. 675). Another participant reported: "My cousin's name is Jihad, I would never yell that out in the airport. I refer to him as Chad" (p. 675). Arab Christian youth who had white sounding names but still "looked" Arab and wanted to differentiate themselves reported that they wore a cross when traveling as to not be mistaken for a Muslim or even to try to dissociate themselves from being seen as Arab. This leads to the next factor of cultural dissociation, which was clothing, especially for those who wore the hijab (head covering) or had family members who wore it.

The next theme found was the use of behavioral management techniques in order to navigate securitization while traveling. One technique reported by participants involved minimizing their use of the Arabic language. For example, one youth reported, "I avoid speaking Arabic despite being with family [and] wait until I am past security. [It's] frustrating that we have to conceal who we are" (p. 676). Another technique involved the altering of behavior or appearance in order to deflect scrutiny of security. For example, male participants reported that they purposely shaved their beards before travel and modified their choice of clothing to blend in more with the mainstream culture or to appear friendlier and unthreatening. The authors noted that these findings were in line with Cainkar (2009) who stated, "Arabs and Muslims in the United States lived with a lurking fear that any impropriety committed at any time in their lives might be brought forth to impugn them. Their behavior needed to meet a standard of perfection reserved for profiled groups: full stops at all stop signs, turn signals on all turns" (p. 4). Finn et al. (2018) comparatively stated that, in their study, "the standard of perfection appears to be the perceived congruity of young people's behavior and dress to White, Anglo-Saxon culture" (p. 676). In addition, the authors found that young Arab women experienced significant forms of racial profiling, which caused them to frequently alter their appearances. Many of them who were Muslim and wore the hijab had to make a conscious effort to minimize scrutiny by engaging in behaviors such as wearing make-up, colorful clothing, and wrapping the hijab in back bun to appear more stylish. For some of these women, the securitization of their identity caused significant distress as security precautions required them to violate their personal sense of bodily integrity and religious standards (Finn et al., 2018).

The third and final theme found was a connection of fear and anxiety to traveling. Many of the Arab youth experienced racism and prejudice directly as a result of traveling. Further, many feared traveling because of the potential discrimination they believed they could experience. One youth reported, "I always get anxious while driving at the American border…[I have] no idea why" (p. 678). The youth expressed a due amount of fear and anxiety about racial profiling and harassment by security personnel while traveling. The participants reported that they made conscious efforts to alter travel plans to avoid scrutiny and even had a list of countries or locations that they would avoid visiting. One participant reported, "Usually for the past years I've had to transit in London, UK or Paris, France…But now, we avoid Europe to be on the safe side, avoid any flight that transits in Europe and specifically search for transits in Turkey as it is similar to Arab [countries]" (p. 678). Finn et al. (2018) asked the Arab youth what they felt was the cause of discrimination and racism. The most common answer was that of the media (Finn et al., 2018). The authors did not examine the effects of these experiences on the Arab youth's development; however, they urged future research to examine the consequences on their well-being.

The experiences of Arab youth in America as a devalued ethnic group warrants investigation of such encounters regarding developmental processes, including ethnic identity, well-being, and, more specifically, self-concept. The literature regarding this group is relatively scarce compared to other ethnic minority groups. The following section presents a narrative review of the literature regarding the relations of discrimination and various aspects of development in adolescents of Arab descent in America. Parts of this narrative review were originally published by Tabbah (2021).[1]

Narrative Review: Discrimination and Developmental Outcomes in Arab American Youth

A literature search was conducted regarding discrimination and developmental processes in adolescents of Arab descent in America. Search terms utilized include Arab American, adolescents, Arab American adolescents, discrimination, well-being, mental health, ethnic identity, self-concept, self-esteem, social identity theory, ecological model, Bronfenbrenner, rejection-identification model, symbolic interaction theory, and stigma hypothesis. Twenty articles were located using the search criteria. Seven articles were excluded due to the age group used in the studies being irrelevant to the current review; while adolescents were included in some of these studies, there was no way to single out their outcomes. One study examined self-concept alone without discrimination factors while another examined ethnic identity and well-being without discrimination factors. Therefore, the final sample for this narrative review consisted of 11 articles. Researchers and practitioners must understand how these experiences potentially influence developmental processes in this group of adolescents.

Self-Concept and Discrimination

Although there is a wealth of research on self-concept and discrimination in various other ethnic minority groups, studies regarding adolescents of Arab descent in America were found to be limited. Two studies were located that examined this relationship. Tabbah, Miranda, and Wheaton (2012) examined different aspects of self-concept in Arab American adolescents in relation to social supports and discrimination in the schools. This was a cross-sectional survey study using a non-random, convenience sample. Snowball sampling was utilized where the authors contacted Arab American organizations around the United States by email and phone, in addition to contacting friends and family members to increase awareness of the study. The total sample included 61 participants ranging between the ages of 12 and 18 years with an average age of 15.3 years. The sample consisted of 28 males

[1]Reprinted by permission from Springer Nature Customer Service Centre GmbH: Springer Nature *Adolescent Research Review* Discrimination and Developmental Processes: Bridging the Research Gap with Adolescents of Arab Descent in America, Rhonda Tabbah, ©2019.

and 33 females. Forty-five (73.8%) were in high school. Participants were 83.6% Muslim, 14.8% Christian, and 1.6% no religious affiliation. The majority of the sample resided in Midwestern states and two-thirds identified as first-generation Americans. Ancestries identified included Palestinian (34.4%), Syrian (23.0%), mixed Arab ancestry (28%), Egyptian (4.9%), Iraqi (4.9%), Jordanian (3.3%), and Yemeni (1.6%). The Self-Perception Profile for Adolescents (SPPA; Harter, 1988) measured three areas of self-concept: Global Self-Worth, Social Acceptance, and Scholastic Competence. The Social Support Scale for Children (SSSC; Harter, 1985) measured participants' self-perceived social support from classmates and teachers. The first author developed a questionnaire to measure concerns that were specific to the study. Participants were asked to self-report whether either they or another Arab student they knew had been "treated badly or differently." If participants answered "Yes" to either question, they were categorized as having experienced discrimination. If they answered "No" to both the questions, they were categorized as not having experienced discrimination. Participants were then asked to elaborate on their experiences and describe what occurred for follow-up purposes. The sample was also compared by school level—middle and high school—to account for possible age group differences.

The authors indicated that half of the sample reported either personal experiences with discrimination, knowing a peer with such exposure, or both. The authors noted that many of the reported experiences by participants were related to students' ethnic and religious identity, such as being called derogatory names, being told to go back to their country, and Muslim females having their head coverings pulled off by classmates. Results suggested that students held overall positive Scholastic Competence, Social Acceptance, and Global Self-Worth, as well as self-perceived classmate and teacher social support. Correlational analyses revealed that Scholastic Competence and teacher support were significantly, positively related to self-reported grade-point average (GPA). Classmate support was significantly, positively related to Scholastic Competence, Social Acceptance, and Global Self-Worth, and negatively related to discrimination. High school students also reported significantly lower Global Self-Worth and Scholastic Competence means than did middle school students. Multiple regression analyses were conducted for each area of self-concept to determine the predictive abilities of variables found to hold significant correlations. Positive perceptions of classmate support, no discrimination, higher GPA, and middle school were found to be significantly predictive of higher Scholastic Competence levels. Higher perceptions of classmate support and middle school status significantly predicted higher Global Self-Worth. Finally, higher perceived classmate support significantly predicted higher Social Acceptance. Results from this study demonstrated that school environment was related to self-concept in this sample of adolescents; more specifically, positive factors related to positive self-concept, whereas negative environmental factors related to negative self-concept.

The limitations of Tabbah et al. (2012) included a cross-sectional nature and the use of a non-random, convenience sample that was small in size. Generalizability was limited, and the use of self-report measures lacked control for response bias and social desirability bias. The study did not take into account demographic factors such as socio-economic status, generational status, acculturation status, nationality/ancestry, and ethnic identity. Also, the ethnic make-up of the schools and communities in which these students resided were not taken into consideration.

In a subsequent piece, Tabbah, Miranda, and Wheaton (2016) investigated areas of self-concept, including physical appearance, athletic competence, behavioral conduct, and close friendship with regard to teacher and classmate support and discrimination in the school system. Similar to the previous study, this survey study was cross-sectional using a non-random, convenience sample obtained by snowball sampling. The sample demographics were identical to Tabbah et al. (2012). Four areas of self-concept were measured using the Self-Perception Profile for Adolescents (SPPA; Harter, 1988): Physical Appearance, Athletic Competence, Behavioral Conduct, and Close Friendship. The Social Support Scale for Children (SSSC; Harter, 1985) was used to measure participants' self-perceived social support from classmates and teachers. The same questionnaire from Tabbah et al. (2012) was utilized to measure discrimination in this study.

Results showed that students had positive self-concept in all areas except for Athletic Competence and Physical Appearance. Perceived classmate and teacher supports were overall positive. Experiences of discrimination personally, vicariously, or both were reported by 31 participants. Examples of reports included being called derogatory names and being treated differently because of the way they physically looked or dressed. Correlational analyses showed that Athletic Competence was significantly, positively related to classmate support and negatively related to gender, with females having significantly lower perceptions than males. Physical Appearance was significantly, positively related to classmate support and negatively related to discrimination, with discrimination experience having lower physical appearance perceptions. The authors rationalized that this finding may have been related to the fact that many adolescents reported being discriminated against because of the way they looked or dressed. Therefore, these experiences may have contributed to the development of adverse thoughts about their physical appearance (Tabbah, Miranda, & Wheaton, 2016). Behavioral Conduct was significantly, positively related to grade point average (GPA) and both classmate and teacher supports. Close Friendship was significantly, positively related to classmate support. Discrimination exposure was negatively associated with perceived classmate support. Teacher support was significantly, positively related to GPA. Multiple regression analyses were conducted for each self-concept model. The Athletic Competence model was significant with higher classmate support and being male predicting higher Athletic Competence perceptions. The Physical Appearance model was significant with no discrimination and higher classmate support predicting higher perceptions of Physical Appearance. The Behavioral Conduct model was significant with higher classmate support, higher teacher support, and higher GPA predicting higher perceptions of Behavior Conduct. Finally, the Close Friendship model was significant with higher classmate support predicting higher perceptions of Close Friendship.

Limitations of Tabbah, Miranda, and Wheaton (2016) were its exploratory nature—as reported by the authors—and the selection process, which limited generalizability of the study. The authors reported having difficulty identifying and contacting Arab American adolescents to participate in the study. Therefore, they utilized snowball sampling to expedite the process. Related to this issue was the relatively small sample size, low response rates, and self-selection. Further limiting generalizability, most of the respondents resided in the Midwestern region of the United States. The authors noted that differences related to religious affiliation and generational status were not able to be examined due to small sample sizes. It was difficult to determine whether being of the Muslim faith was a contributing factor of discrimination experiences. Furthermore, in terms of generational status, the second- and third-generation adolescents may have been less prone to discrimination than the first-generation adolescents depending on their acculturation experiences. Finally, the nature of the discrimination questionnaire did not allow for the reporting of frequency of experiences and only focused on the school setting.

Ethnic Identity and Discrimination

Studies examining the relationship between ethnic identity and discrimination with adolescents of Arab descent in America were relatively limited with inconsistent results. Seven articles were located that investigated this process. Flanagan, Syvertsen, Gill, Gallay, and Cumsille (2009) examined the relationship between ethnic background, experiences of prejudice, and ethnic awareness with Arab American, African American, Latino American, and European American youth. The data for this study was collected prior to September 11, 2011 during a relatively calm period in the United States, as reported by the authors. The sample was obtained from three communities in the Midwest and Northeastern regions of the United States by advertising through the school systems. The sample consisted of 1096 adolescents from African (115), Arab (115), Latino (127), and European (749) ethnic backgrounds. Ages ranged from 11 to 18 years. The Arab sample was found to be the oldest group followed by European, African, and Latino students. The sample was 53% female. The majority of the samples of African and European American were third generation or higher, while the majority of the Latino and Arab American samples were first and second generation. Arab and Latino American adolescents reported significantly lower parental education than did African and European American adolescents. Due to the demographic differences found by ethnic group, the authors utilized age, gender, and parental education as covariates in statistical analyses. All measures used in this study were based on self-report. For ethnic self-identification, participants were asked to choose from a list that best described their ancestry. Ethnic awareness was measured by asking students how aware they were about their racial, ethnic, or cultural identity. They were to choose either "very aware" or "not very aware." The authors measured experiences of prejudice by asking adolescents to respond "yes" or "no" to the question, "Have you or someone close to you ever faced prejudice?" and, then, asking them to elaborate on their experience. Chi-square tests were used to test for differences between ethnic groups in their ethnic awareness and experiences of prejudice and to test—by ethnic group—the relationship between adolescents' ethnic awareness and whether or not they had experienced prejudice.

Results showed a significant relationship between adolescents' ethnic background and their ethnic awareness. For both African and Arab American students, 66% of them reported that they or someone they knew had experienced prejudice, compared to 48% of Latino and 47% of European American students. The majority of the discriminatory acts occurred in schools and informal settings, such as sporting events or hanging out with friends. For Latino, Arab, and African American adolescents, restaurants, stores, and banks were also likely settings for experiencing discrimination. The authors observed a statistically significant relationship between ethnic awareness and experiences of prejudice for European and Latino Americans but not for Arab or African American adolescents. Flanagan et al. (2009) suggested that this might have been because most participants from the latter two groups reported experiencing prejudice, therefore, limiting the power to detect true relationships.

Limitations to Flanagan et al. (2009) included a cross-sectional design and reliance on self-report to collect data. The scales used on measures contained relatively few items, which likely affected the internal consistency of those measures. Furthermore, only one aspect of ethnic identity, ethnic awareness, was measured. Since the study only measured one time point, the authors were not able to examine changes in ethnic awareness and identity over time and in response to experiences in different contexts.

Ahmed, Kia-Keating, and Tsai (2011) investigated the role of socio-cultural adversities and cultural resources in terms of their direct impact on psychological distress in Arab American adolescents. Socio-cultural adversities consisted of perceived discrimination and acculturative stress. Cultural resources included ethnic identity, religious coping, and religious support. Psychological distress encompassed internalizing and externalizing symptoms, depression, and anxiety. The main purpose of the study was to test a risk and resilience model using structural equation modeling that delineates the relationships between these socio-cultural adversities, cultural resources, and psychological distress. The final sample consisted of 240 (124 male and 116 female) Arab American high school students ranging in age from 13 to 18 years. The sample was recruited from a high school that was predominantly Arab American and situated in one of the largest Arab American communities in the United States. The majority of the sample identified as Muslim (204), while three were Christian, 20 identified as Atheist or did not answer, and 13 reported ethnicity instead of religious affiliation. Parents were asked to provide information regarding socioeconomic status, refugee status, and family history of mental illness. Adolescents were asked to self-report on age, gender, grade, religion, generational status, and personal mental health history. A modified version of the Perceived Racism Scale-Child (Nyborg, 2000) assessed perceived discrimination. This measure was originally developed for African American populations, so the authors substituted "Black" with "Arab." The Societal, Attitudinal, Environmental, and Familial Acculturative Stress Scale (SAFE; Padilla, Wagatsuma, & Lindholm, 1985) measured acculturative stress. The Multigroup Ethnic Identity Measure (MEIM; Phinney, 1992) measured aspects of ethnic identity, including ethnic affirmation, belongingness, pride, and participation in ethnic group related activities. The Brief Religious Coping Measure (Pargament, Smith, Koenig, & Perez, 1998) assessed religious coping, with modifications of items that included the word "God" to be changed to "God or Allah." The Religious Support Scale (Fiala, Bjorck, & Gorsuch, 2002) measured religious support, with similar modifications of the word "God" to "God or Allah" and "church" or "congregation" to "mosque/church" or "mosque/congregation." The Child Behavior Checklist-Youth Self Report (Achenbach & Rescorla, 2001) assessed internalizing and externalizing symptoms. The Center for Epidemiologic Studies Depression Scale (Radloff, 1977) measured frequency of depressive symptoms, while the State Trait Anxiety Inventory (Spielberger, 1983) assessed situational and stable aspects of anxiety.

Correlational analyses showed significant correlations between generational status and ethnic identity and religious coping; specifically, being of an earlier generational status was related to greater ethnic identity and increased religious coping. Female adolescents were more likely to be of an earlier generational status, more likely to report increased religious support and ethnic identity, and reported fewer externalizing symptoms. Increased perceived racism was related to increased acculturative stress, increased depression, anxiety, internalizing and externalizing symptoms, and less religious support. Higher acculturative stress was related to increased levels of depression and internalizing and externalizing symptoms. Increased ethnic identity levels were correlated with higher religious support and coping, as well as fewer depression, anxiety, and internalizing and externalizing symptoms. Religious support was negatively related with depression, anxiety, and internalizing and externalizing symptoms, and positively correlated with religious coping. Higher levels of religious coping were associated with lower levels of depression, anxiety, and internalizing and externalizing symptoms. All psychological distress measures were significantly, positively correlated. In terms of the structural equation model, the authors utilized gender and generational status as covariates in the model. Severity of psychological distress was predicted by two separate, direct pathways. The first pathway demonstrated that greater socio-cultural adversity was related to more psychological distress. The second pathway showed that increased cultural resources were related to lower psychological distress. Further, 97% of the variance in psychological distress was explained by socio-cultural adversity, cultural resources, generational status, and gender. The authors conducted post hoc analyses to determine moderation abilities of cultural resources on psychological distress in the face of socio-cultural adversity. However, results suggested that there was no moderation of cultural resources on the effects of socio-cultural adversity on psychological distress. In contrast to the rejection-identification model, the authors found that ethnic identity was not correlated with perceived racism nor was it a protective factor in the psychological distress of adolescents who perceived racism.

Limitations of Ahmed et al. (2011) included a cross-sectional design, which prevented the authors from measuring causal directionality of cultural resources and socio-cultural adversities on psychological distress. Further, students were self-selected for participation and the authors suggested that students who experienced more adversities may have been more prone to participating in the study. Generalizability was also limited due to the sampling taking place in a single community and also due to the sample being primarily Muslim. The latter does not allow reflection on the experiences of Arab Christian counterparts.

Kumar, Warnke, and Karabenick (2014) examined the identities of Arab descent male adolescents in relation to their ethnicity, religion, nationality, and current contexts, including public perceptions, experiences of discrimination, and stereotype awareness. This was a qualitative study that utilized focus groups with 79 eighth-grade male students that were systematically selected based on a random sampling of students stratified by ethnicity, gender, and primary language spoken at home as identified in school records. Because US census records classify individuals from Arab ancestry as white, the authors stratified white by language spoken at home to distinguish Arab from other students. All participants were either born in the United States or living there since early childhood. The study was conducted in seven economically diverse middle schools in the Midwestern region of the United States. Four of the seven schools were majority Arab or Arab American. In one school, Arab/Arab Americans made up half of the population, while European Americans were one-third of the population. In the remaining two schools, the majority of the students consisted of European Americans. The focus group interview protocol included questions regarding the nature of intergroup contact in and out of school; feelings of inclusion and exclusion; perceptions of stereotyping and discrimination in both school and societal contexts; political consciousness; experiences associated with attending schools inside and outside ethnic enclaves; expressions of gender-specific cultural expectations; contextual and phenomenological saliency of masculine and aggressive male Arab identities; and endorsement of pan-Arab, Arab-American, assimilated American national, and religious identities.

Results showed that identity negotiations in this group of Arab descent males were complicated due to their childhood years being dominated by post-9/11 public anger, prejudice, and discrimination. The authors identified three major themes that emerged through the focus group interviews. First, adolescents' understanding of masculinity was interconnected with their religious and cultural identity. Arab descent male identity was influenced by the prominent US perceptions of Arab males as aggressive and Arab females as submissive. However, the authors did find variability among the participants' interpretations of religion, nationality, and male–female counter roles and the importance of these factors in forming their masculine identity. For example, while some viewed the Muslim identity as prominent, others showed preference for a sectarian identity. A student who identified himself as Christian expressed a more assimilated identity and would distance himself during more heated arguments of the interview. In addition, the authors found that the interaction of religion with masculinity was more prominent in Muslim participants than with Christian or secular participants. The authors suggested that this variability spoke to the heterogeneity that exists among Arab Americans.

Second, the authors identified an effect of heightened political consciousness and stereotype awareness associated with Arab American males on their social identity. The authors reported high levels of political consciousness and comprehension of US policies in the Middle East. Many of the students discussed the war in the Middle East and the impact on their lives and the lives of people living in that region. They also demonstrated a heightened political awareness during discussions regarding the role of the media in developing perceptions of world events and stereotypes of Arabs as well as discussions on how they navigated these complicated issues. Discussions revealed the level of alienation these students have experienced from mainstream American culture. For example, one student stated, "They won't put anything good about us on the news" (p. 32). Students from the predominantly white school reported feeling disenfranchised because their personal and group experiences were not valued by their peers and teachers. The authors suggested that such experiences may potentially affect the strength of Arab descent adolescents' identification with their in-group and distrust of outgroup members and effect their feelings about residing in a country that is—in particular situations—at war with their countries of origin. Students also showed heightened stereotype awareness, especially of the aggressive Arab male stereotype. Students reported times where they felt misjudged and unwelcomed in the United States. They expressed feeling anger, frustration, and anxiety as a result. Some of the incidents involved hostile and violent encounters outside their neighborhoods from members of the dominant society who did not know the students personally. One student stated, "Their [non-Arab classmates] parents will be watching the news … and they'll [non-Arab students] come to school saying 'you're a terrorist, you went and bombed this and that'" (p. 33). This leads to the next stereotype awareness theme among the students, which was the terrorist stereotype, often linked to Arab American male identity. Then, the authors identified four different coping strategies used by students in the face of perceived stereotyping, prejudice, and discrimination: reactive, denial, passive, and positive/transformative. The authors defined reactive coping strategies as negative, aggressive, and ineffective responses to discrimination experiences. Denial coping was defined as refusing to acknowledge the existence of any discrimination even when it is directed at them personally, which occurred to protect their self-worth. Passive coping refers to internalizing the experience and becoming anxious and/or depressed because they felt powerless over the situation. Those who found ways to counter prejudice directed toward them through seeking supportive and open discussions demonstrated positive/transformative coping. Participants across all schools reported the experiences of their family members and community as targets of prejudice and discrimination as a result of such stigma and stereotypes.

Third, the authors identified a theme of a sliding social identity where they found multifaceted social identities that changed in content and prominence depending on the topic of discussion and how it unraveled in the group. For example, where a participant might use the term "we" in reference to Americans in one context, they might change to the term "they" to identify Americans and "we" to identify Arabs in another context. The authors also reported that the salience of social identities depended on the cultural diversity within the school framework. For example, students who attended the more culturally diverse schools were required to confront and negotiate the meaning of their social identities within their own groups and their perceptions of intergroup relations in school. The authors found greater intragroup variability in the identity negotiations of students attending these schools. The authors reported evidence that in schools where intergroup and intercultural contact was common, participants' self-identification ranged on the assimilation continuum from desire to assimilate as an American to a strong Arab identity that denounced American status. On the contrary, students attending predominantly Arab/Arab American schools with less intercultural contact stated more comfort and a strong sense of belonging to the school and the Muslim, Arab American community. These students did not have to battle with the daily exposure to discrimination or prejudice. The authors concluded that, for these adolescents, the school and community buffered against societal stereotyping, prejudice, and discrimination. In addition, these adolescents identified themselves based on country of origin in order to preserve optimal distinctiveness.

In conclusion, the authors found that the devalued status of these male adolescents of Arab descent in society reinforced their identities and, in the face of social and political adversities, reinforced a need to be surrounded by their in-group members (Kumar et al., 2014). Limitations were not cited by Kumar et al. (2014); however, while the randomized selection of participants was a strength, the focus-group nature limited generalizability of results to the sample. Also, the cross-sectional nature limited any detection of changes in identity over time and related to different social adversities and political conditions.

Tabbah, Wheaton, and Miranda (2015) examined ethnic identity in relation to discrimination experiences specific to the school system. This was a cross-sectional survey study using a non-random, convenience sample. Snowball sampling was utilized where the authors contacted Arab American organizations around the United States by email and phone, in addition to contacting friends and family members to increase awareness of the study. The authors reported a 28.3% response rate with 68 of 240 surveys returned. Seven of the 68 did not meet eligibility criteria or did not complete the forms correctly. The final sample consisted of 61 (28 male and 33 female) respondents ranging in age from 12 to 18 years. The majority of the participants identified themselves as Muslim (83.6%), while 14.8% identified themselves as Christian, and one reported no religious affiliation. Participants largely resided in the Midwestern region of the United States. Two-thirds of the sample were first generation. Ancestry included Palestinian (34.4%), mixed Arab ancestry (28%), Syrian (23%), Egyptian (4.9%), Jordanian (3.3%), and Yemeni (1.6%). The authors used the Multigroup Ethnic Identity Measure (MEIM; Phinney, 1992) to assess ethnic identity, including ethnic identity search and affirmation/belonging. The ethnic identity search subscale measures the degree to which individuals explore, learn about, and become involved in their ethnic group. Affirmation/belonging measures feelings of attachment, sense of belonging, and commitment to one's ethnic group. In order to measure experiences of discrimination, the first author developed a questionnaire to measure specific experiences in the school system. Participants were asked to self-report if either they or another Arab student they knew had been treated badly or differently. Two questions were asked, the first one questioned personal experiences while the second one questioned vicarious experiences. Based on the answers, the authors categorized the students into four different groups. Students who answered "No" to both the questions were categorized under "No discrimination." Students who answered "Yes" to either personal experiences or knowing another Arab with experiences were labeled under either "Discrimination of self" or "Discrimination of others," respectively. Students who answered "Yes" to both the questions were placed under "Multiple experiences."

Results showed that 31 participants reported experiencing some form of discrimination in the schools: nine endorsed personal experience, seven reported knowing others who were discriminated against, and 15 reported having both the experiences. The remaining 30 reported no experiences, some of whom noted that they believed it was because they were not recognized as Arab. The authors found that ethnic identity search was significantly, positively related to both "Discrimination of self" and "Discrimination of others." Affirmation/belonging was positively related to "Discrimination of self" only. In terms of demographic variables, gender was not significant; however, age was negatively related to affirmation/belonging with increasing age corresponding to decreased affirmation/belonging scores. Omnibus ANOVAs were conducted on each ethnic identity subscale. The "Multiple experiences" group held the highest means on both ethnic identity search and affirmation/belonging subscales. The omnibus ANOVA was statistically significant on both subscales. Furthermore, Tukey's post hoc analysis indicated that those in the "Multiple experiences" group had significantly higher mean scores than those in the "No discrimination" group on both ethnic identity search and affirmation/belonging measures. No other post hoc comparisons were found to be significant. The authors speculated that the ability to cope with prejudice might depend on how pervasive an individual perceives discrimination to be against his or her community; a single experience of discrimination may be coped with differently than multiple instances or pervasive discrimination (Branscombe, Schmitt, & Harvey, 1999).

Limitations of Tabbah et al. (2015) included snowball sampling, a cross-sectional design, and a relatively small sample size. The study sample was not considered representative of the Arab American population, as the sample majority was Muslim and the Arab American population majority is actually Christian (Amer & Kayyali, 2016). The authors also reported difficulty in the selection process due to complications with identifying Arab American participants. Therefore, the sample had to be selected purposively, which also limited the generalizability of the results. Important factors such as generational status were not taken into consideration due to small group sizes.

In a subsequent study, Tabbah, Chung, and Miranda (2016) utilized the sample and methodology cited in Tabbah et al. (2015) to investigate self-concept with ethnic identity and discrimination in the school system. For the purposes of the analysis to compare religious differences, the authors removed the one participant with no religious affiliation. Therefore, the final sample consisted of 60 (27 male and 33 female) participants. Forty-one students reported being first-generation, 15 were second-generation, and four were third generation. For generational comparison, the second and third generations were combined into one group. The researchers utilized two subscales of ethnic identity from the MEIM (Phinney, 1992), which included affirmation/belonging and ethnic search. The authors utilized the same discrimination questionnaire from Tabbah et al. (2015). Based on the answers, the authors categorized the students into two groups. Students who answered "No" to both questions were categorized under "No discrimination." Students who answered "Yes" to personal experiences or knowing another Arab with experiences, or both were labeled under "Discrimination." The subscales Global Self-Worth and Scholastic Competence were examined using the SPPA (Harter, 1988), as the authors considered these most relevant to school experiences.

Results showed that 31 students reported experiencing some form of discrimination. Ethnic identity scores were considered high overall for both the subscales. Self-concept scores for both Global Self-Worth and Scholastic Competence were high as well. Mean differences for ethnic search and affirmation/belonging were not significant by gender nor by generational status. A significant mean difference was found in ethnic search between Muslim and Christian groups, with Christians holding significantly higher mean scores than Muslims; however, no significant difference was found with affirmation/belonging and religion. Ethnic search was significantly higher in the discrimination group as compared to the no discrimination group. The authors found no significant differences between these two groups for affirmation/belonging. They also found no significant group differences in the examination of Global Self-Worth and Scholastic Competence, with the exception of a borderline significant difference in discrimination groups where the discrimination group held lower perceptions of Scholastic Competence than the no discrimination group. Correlational analyses revealed significant negative relations between age and both Scholastic Competence and Global Self-Worth: as age increased self-concept scores decreased. Age was also negatively associated with affirmation/belonging; with increasing age, there was decreasing perceptions of affirmation/belonging. Scholastic Competence was significantly, positively related to self-reported GPA and affirmation/belonging. Affirmation/belonging was significantly, positively related to Global Self-Worth and ethnic search. The open-ended questionnaires for discrimination were analyzed for common themes revealing the following: stereotypes of Arabs being Muslim, stereotypes as radical and dangerous, stereotypes as inferior or other. Multiple regression analyses were conducted and two models of self-concept were developed including Global Self-Worth and Scholastic Competence. The Global Self-Worth model was significant with affirmation/belonging and age having significant predictive abilities. Higher affirmation/belonging and younger age predicted higher Global Self-Worth. The authors observed a medium effect size for this model. The Scholastic Competence model was significant with discrimination, age, affirmation/belonging, and self-reported GPA holding significant predictive abilities. Younger students with no discrimination experience, higher affirmation/belonging, and higher GPA predicted higher levels of Scholastic Competence. The authors observed a large effect size for this model.

Limitations of Tabbah, Chung, and Miranda (2016) included a cross-sectional design, relatively small sample size, and the use of purposive selection with the use of volunteers due to difficulties identifying Arab American participants. While generational status was taken into consideration, the sample sizes may have been too small to detect any true differences. Also, due to small sample sizes, differences in Arab nationality were not able to be examined. The study sample was not considered representative of the Arab American population regarding nationality and religious affiliation; specifically, the sample majority was Muslim and the Arab American population majority is Christian (Amer & Kayyali, 2016). These issues along with purposive sampling limited the generalizability of the results.

Kumar, Seay, and Karabenick (2015) examined risk and protective factors related to identity negotiation and adjustment of recent immigrant Arab adolescents in the United States residing in ethnic enclaves. The authors conducted focus-group interviews with 45 eighth grade immigrant Arab early adolescents from four middle schools located within ethnic enclaves. These schools were considered majority Arab/Arab American. The sample consisted of Yemeni (60%), Iraqi (15%), and Lebanese (9%) backgrounds with a small percentage from other unidentified Arab countries. Twenty-five students were male and 20 were female. Participants were selected by random sampling of the eighth-grade students stratified by ethnicity, primary language spoken at home, and years in the United States as reported in school records. Students had to be residing in the United States for 3 years or less. The authors further stratified the sample by gender when possible and reported that this process ensured homogeneity of the focus-group participants. Random selection was conducted by selecting every fifth or third student on the roster. The authors asked questions regarding perceptions of the school context, including teachers' cultural sensitivity and culturally responsive teaching; feelings of inclusion or exclusion and dissonance in community and school context; perceptions of stereotyping and discrimination; media depiction of Arabs; and contextual and phenomenological saliency of immigrant, national, religious, and refugee identities.

Results showed that immigrants' transition from their country of origin to host culture, acculturation process, and identity negotiations were interconnected with their social, cultural, and physical contexts. The authors found that these adolescents' identities were also influenced by their experiences prior to immigration and by the immigration process. Several themes were identified within these processes. First, participants' immigration experiences varied according to conditions in their origin countries. For example, some of the immigrant adolescents were displaced during the first Iraq war and resettled in the United States. Some of these students were born and resided in refugee camps for several years before resettling in the United States, while others lived in other Middle Eastern countries before resettlement. Consequently, residing in an ethnic enclave with other Iraqi adolescents with similar refugee experiences created a symbolic Iraqi identity and developed feelings of relatedness among these adolescent participants. The authors speculated that being surrounded by adolescents with similar immigration experiences likely served as a protective factor to their psychological well-being. In addition, the authors found that whether or not these adolescents' immigration was voluntary influenced their desire for integration into mainstream society. Specifically, Yemeni students who reported voluntary immigration of their parents for economic and educational advancement also expressed more readily the desire to become part of American mainstream society while still being committed to traditional cultural and Islamic practices.

Second, students felt that the ethnic enclave was a place where they belonged, where their cultural dress and behavior were valued, and where they were protected from angry looks and discriminatory behavior. However, interestingly enough, these adolescents did not express anger or frustration with negative public images of Arabs as compared to Arab/Arab American students that participated in a larger study by these authors (Kumar et al., 2014). The authors speculated that these adolescents' view of America was influenced by their everyday experiences in the ethnic enclave; specifically, they viewed America to be supportive of Arab cultures.

Third, the quality of reception of these immigrant adolescents was related to the local neighborhood and school. Results showed that resettlement in an ethnic enclave helped these students to maintain their religious and cultural values and norms. The authors reported that this relationship seemed to ameliorate stress involved with immigration and resettlement. In addition, the need for religious commitment seemed to stem from a need to develop social bonds to replace those that were lost by immigration. Immigrant Arab adolescent females did not feel the same safety and support outside of the ethnic enclave. For example, they felt overly conscious of their distinctive appearance in terms of dressing modestly (i.e., wearing hijab, a head covering) and their immigrant status when they were outside the limits of the ethnic enclave. Some of these female adolescents expressed perceptions of anger from others that was prompted by their dress. The authors concluded that while residing in ethnic enclaves sheltered these adolescents from prejudice and discrimination, experiences with mainstream society increased their awareness of being unwelcomed immigrants.

Fourth, the authors found that neighborhood schools in ethnic enclaves were better equipped than non-ethnic enclave schools to serve immigrant Arab adolescents for two reasons: first, the student body in ethnic enclave schools was primarily Arab/Arab American and reflected the national and religious demographics of the surrounding neighborhood. Therefore, this was a source of comfort for these adolescents. Second, the school staff in ethnic enclave schools—regardless of their own cultural background—were more culturally competent to meet the needs of their student body. Consequently, these factors were identified as protective factors by the authors.

However, there were downfalls of ethnic enclave schools unique to these immigrant adolescents, which leads to the next two themes: the immigrant adolescents expressed an unexpected hierarchy of status based upon nationality within the ethnic enclave schools. Students reported being rejected by Arab students who emigrated from other countries in the Middle East. Both established Arab/Arab American and newly immigrant students maintained a distinct identity based on their national identity. Students demonstrated an awareness of their own group relative to other Arab groups. An example presented was that a Lebanese student described Yemeni students as "smelly" (p. 207). Students also reported that boys would self-segregate based on national identity and would bully out-group members. The authors concluded that the acculturation process for this group of immigrant Arabs was further complicated by their identification with the pan-Arab community, in addition to disparities between mainstream and heritage circumstances and cultures. Another risk factor identified by the authors was the risk of rejection and identity confusion in the school context. The authors reported that students sometimes felt invalidated by their teachers and peers as they would challenge the meaning and value of immigrants' cultural and religious identity. Cultural and religious values that were the norm in their origin countries were demeaned and ridiculed among both mainstream peers and well-established Arab/Arab American peers. The authors reported that cultural dissonance was further complicated through taunting by Arab descent adolescent males including name-calling, discrimination, and rejection. Female participants were also rejected because they maintained their traditional way of dressing. In addition, when these students complained to staff about their experiences, they were ignored. Students also felt rejected due to their lack of English fluency. Finally, conflict and confusion were created for both male and female participants due to misunderstanding and perceived misinterpretation of behaviors by teachers. The authors speculated that these reactions may have been fueled by teachers' biased views mirroring societal negative stereotypes and prejudices of the Arab community.

In terms of limitations, none were cited by Kumar et al. (2015). While the randomized selection of participants was a strength, the focus-group nature and the selection of participants from one community limited generalizability of results to the sample at hand. Additionally, the cross-sectional nature limited any detection of changes in identity over time and related to different social adversities and political conditions.

More recently, Najjar, Naser, and Clonan-Roy (2019) conducted a qualitative focus group study with Arab American early college students and community dwellers where participants were asked to reflect on their primary school experiences with discrimination and how this related to their identity development. A sample of 21 (ten female), first-generation Arab American youth participated in this study with ages ranging from 18 to 23 years. All participants were either born in an Arab country or had at least one parent who was born in an Arab country. Arab heritage of participants included Palestinian, Lebanese, Syrian, Kuwaiti, and Saudi Arabian. Twelve identified as Muslim and nine as Christian. Convenience, snowball sampling was used to recruit participants. Questions reported by the authors were related to school-based support and discrimination. Participants were first asked what being Arab American meant to them, and the remaining questions focused on school experiences.

Results from qualitative analyses showed that there were three mechanisms by which the school setting distinctively impacted Arab heritage students' acculturation processes and subsequent identity negotiations in high school. The first mechanism was peer and teacher discrimination. The youth who experienced discrimination in school responded by either distancing themselves from their cultural heritage or distancing themselves from non-Arab individuals. The authors also reported that teacher-initiated discrimination may have uniquely impacted student sense of belonging in the school setting. The second mechanism was the treatment of Arab history and culture in the school curriculum. The authors found that a lack of representation, misrepresentation, or exclusively negative representation of Arab history and culture in school curriculum was a source of acculturative stress for these Arab heritage youth. This either caused students to distance themselves from their cultural heritage or to engage in cognitive and emotional exertion to ameliorate the representation of Arab culture and history presented in the curriculum. The third mechanism was the allowance for student cultural expression through broader school structures. The authors reported that while these students engaged in cognitive and emotional labor to educate others about their culture, formal opportunities for cultural expression permitted within the school setting reduced the barriers to participating in this endeavor. In terms of their identity, for each of these three mechanisms described, students reported either distancing themselves from, or leaning into their ethnic identity as a coping mechanism to feelings of discrimination, exclusion, or silencing (Najjar et al., 2019).

Limitations of Najjar et al. (2019) included snowball sampling within one university and geographic region within the United States, which limited generalization of the results. Also, the study involved collecting retroactive data from individuals who had graduated from high school and were either currently involved in undergraduate studies or had earned a bachelor's degree.

Well-Being and Discrimination

Only two studies were located that examined general well-being and discrimination in Arab American youth. Albdour, Lewin, Kavanaugh, Hong, and Wilson (2017) conducted a qualitative study with ten Arab American adolescents who were victims of bullying to describe their experiences and related stress. The authors examined bullying situations where these adolescents were victimized, how they felt when bullied, and how they coped with stress and bullying. Ten Arab American adolescents (six females and four males) between the ages of 14 and 16 years were recruited from a well-known Arab community center in a Midwestern state that provides social and health services to Arab American immigrants. Eight of the adolescents were born in the United States, while two were born in Iraq. Countries of origin included Iraq (6), Lebanon (2), and Palestine (2). Participants were interviewed in their homes to promote feelings of safety when sharing their experiences. The authors asked questions to obtain a description of the bullying events, how they felt when bullied, and how overwhelmed they felt when bullied. They asked questions about the adolescent's perceived stress that were derived from the Perceived Stress Scale (Cohen, Kamarck, & Mermelstein, 1983). Finally, the authors asked questions about how long the adolescents felt that way and what helped them cope with their feelings.

When examining the types of bullying experienced, results showed that all participants were verbally bullied by their peers by use of hurtful words or comments, making fun of them, yelling at them, or making threats to them. All participants also experienced being excluded by their peers in group projects and other activities. The adolescents reported feeling rejected or unwelcomed. Six participants reported being physically bullied. Only two indicated being cyberbullied through phone messages. Results showed that bullying was more frequent among the boys in the sample, with three of the four boys reporting severe experiences compared to only one girl.

In examination of reasons for being bullied, all but one of the participants indicated that the bullying was related to their race and ethnicity. Half of the participants reported that the only reason they were bullied was due to "being Arabic" (p. 1575). Peers used hateful and racist words or comments against them, such as "terrorist," "boarder," "go back to your country," and "towel head" (p. 1575). Several of the participants were bullied because of their names, which represent their Arab and Islamic backgrounds. One of the participants changed his name because it was associated with a well-known terrorist and students would shout at him, "He is a terrorist… he is going to terrorize the school… he has a bomb" (p. 1575). Further, several participants were bullied because they spoke Arabic or were not proficient in English. All female participants who wore a head covering were bullied because of their scarves. Peers would call them "towel head" or "scarfy," or make comments such as, "Do you shower with this" or "Are you bald?" (p. 1576). Five participants reported that, in addition to being bullied because of their race and ethnicity, they were also bullied because of a health problem, being overweight, or having a social disadvantage.

Results from examining the context of bullying indicated that bullying happened early in their lives in elementary school. However, most of their bullying experiences were recent and happened within the last 2 years. Most participants described verbal bullying as being the worst with only one indicating that physical bullying was the most hurtful. Occurrences of bullying typically happened within the school context or a school-related area or facility. Two participants reported experiences during a field trip outside of school and two others experienced bullying at the mall.

Next, Albdour et al. (2017) examined stress levels experienced from bullying. All of the participants except for one reported feeling very stressed and anxious for various reasons when they were bullied. Four reported feeling stressed because they did not want to confront the bullies or did not know what to do or say to them. Four reported that they felt a lot of pressure and kept thinking about the bullying situation all the time. Three of the participants cried at home after being bullied. Some reported that they had physical symptoms because their stress levels were so high. One even sought anxiety medication, while another reported that the stress from being bullied was one of the reasons she developed a skin disease.

In terms of feelings when bullied, a wide range of negative feelings were reported by the participants, with the most common being feeling upset, sad, angry, overwhelmed, and hurt. This was prevalent with both male and female participants. In addition, most of the participants reported feeling like they lost control over things that were important to them, especially school work and performance. They reported feeling distracted and having difficulty with concentration in school as they were consumed with bullying all the time and were not able to focus. Other participants reported having school avoidance to prevent having to confront the bullies. Four reported losing any confidence they had in how they handled other life problems.

The final area of examination regarded the adolescents' coping strategies. In terms of coping behaviors, most of the participants reported that they will never forget their bullying experiences and that it took them a long time to stop thinking about what happened. Six reported that it took months or years to cope; others reported days or weeks, with the severely bullied participants taking longer to cope. The adolescents reported poor coping behaviors at the time the bullying occurred and did not develop more useful strategies until later. Ineffective coping strategies included over eating or crying while more effective strategies included exercising and sports. When it came to available support and resources, the majority of participants reported having family that provided relief and support. Only one participant reported having a teacher to talk to that was helpful. Conversely, four of the adolescents reported that their teachers did not stop the bullying and even blamed the victims for being bullied. Further, two participants reported being bullied and discriminated against by their teachers. Eight participants indicated that they were bullied by adults in school in addition to being bullied by their peers. For example, one participant reported:

> Just because I asked the teacher what did he means by one word that he said, I told him can you please express this word in another way, he pushed me down to the corner of the room and start yelling at me after class. He yelled at me for 15 min straight. (p. 1580)

Limitations of Albdour et al. (2017) included a small number of participants from one geographical area, which limited generalizability of the results. In addition, the results relied on self-report with no confirmation from other sources, which the authors note may have increased the credibility of their findings (Albdour et al., 2017). Finally, the authors did not account for other factors that may influence stress levels that might have affected their findings (Albdour et al., 2017).

Goforth, Oka, Leong, and Denis (2014) examined acculturation, acculturative stress, religiosity, and psychological adjustment in Muslim Arab American adolescents. Perceived discrimination was examined as part of acculturative stress in this study. Research shows that perceived discrimination, acculturative stress, and mental health are strongly associated (Ahmed et al., 2011). The authors recruited participants from a health clinic that serves a large Arab American population in a large Midwestern city. A total of 128 Muslim Arab American adolescents participated in the study with ages ranging between 11 and 21 years. The authors indicated that some participants did not report their age or gender, which left the study with missing data. Twenty-eight participants were in middle school, 54 were in high school, and 25 were post-high school. Twenty-nine participants were born in the United States, while 96 were born elsewhere.

The authors used the Vancouver Index of Acculturation (VIA; Ryder, Alden, & Paulhus, 2000), a self-report measure using a bidimensional model of acculturation to measure acculturation status, or degree to which an individual displays characteristics or behaviors associated with each culture. Specifically, the measure holds a Heritage scale (VIA-H) and an American scale (VIA-A). The Societal, Academic, Familial, and Environmental Acculturative Stress Scale: Children's Version (SAFE-C; Chavez, Moran, Reid, & Lopez, 1997) measured various aspects of acculturative stress. The General Social Stress scale measures general stressors that all children may experience regardless of ethnicity. The Process-Oriented Stress subscale measures the process of acculturation. The Perceived Discrimination Stress subscale measures perceptions of discrimination. The authors administered the Brief Multidimensional Measure of Religiosity/Spirituality to measure religiosity (Pargament, 1999), including Organizational Religiousness, Private Religious Practices, and Overall Spirituality and Religiousness. These domains were highly intercorrelated. Therefore, the authors summed the scale scores and computed a Religiosity Composite. The Reynolds Short Form A of the Marlowe-Crowne Social Desirability Scale (Crowne & Marlowe, 1960) measured social desirability to minimize response bias. Results from this measure indicated that there was not a high degree of social desirability in the participants' responses. Finally, an English or Arabic version of the Youth Self-Report (YSR; Achenbach & Rescorla, 2001) measured psychological adjustment through two scales: Social Competence and Total Problems.

Correlational analyses showed significant negative correlations between length of time living in the United States and all three acculturative stress measures: process-oriented stress, perceived discrimination stress, and global stress. Significant positive correlations were found between American orientation on the acculturation scale (VIA-A) and perceived discrimination stress and global stress. Heritage culture orientation (VIA-H) was significantly negatively correlated with YSR-Total Problems but not YSR-Competence. The authors speculate that this self-reported orientation to Arab culture was associated with lower self-reported psychological problems but not higher or lower competence (Goforth et al., 2014). Global stress was positively associated with YSR-Total Problems and negatively associated with YSR-Competence. More specifically, adolescents who reported higher global stress related to acculturation also reported more psychological problems and less overall competence. Further, it is worth noting that perceived discrimination stress was significantly positively related to YSR-Total Problems and negatively related to YSR-Competence.

Goforth et al. (2014) performed a series of simultaneous regressions to examine the predictive ability of a variety of models. The predictive ability of age, gender, religiosity, and length of time in the United States on the acculturation variables of Heritage (VIA-H) and American (VIA-A) scales was examined. The VIA-A model was not significant, whereas the VIA-H model was with religiosity holding the strongest predictive ability. Participants who endorsed higher religiosity also endorsed a stronger orientation to their heritage culture.

The same variables of age, gender, religiosity, and length of time in the United States were examined on acculturative stress variables from the SAFE-C, including General Social Stress, Perceived Discrimination, and Process-Oriented Stress. The General Social Stress model was significant with age, gender, religiosity, and length of time in the United States all having significant predictive ability. Increased age, religiosity, and length of time in the United States, predicted less General Social Stress. The Perceived Discrimination model was also significant with gender, religiosity, and length of time in the United States holding significant effects. Increased religiosity and length of time in the United States predicted lower Perceived Discrimination Stress. The Process-Oriented Stress model was significant with religiosity holding the strongest predictive ability. Increased religiosity predicted lower Process-Oriented Stress.

The final set of regression models examined the predictive ability of VIA-A, VIA-H, and SAFE-C on psychological adjustment variables of the YSR-Total Problems and YSR-Competence. The YSR-Total Problems model was significant with VIA-H and SAFE-C being significant predictors. Higher VIA-H levels predicted lower Total Problems and higher SAFE-C predicted higher Total Problems. Specifically, a high Arab culture heritage orientation predicted lower psychological problems, and higher acculturative stress predicted more psychological problems. The YSR-Competence model was also significant with VIA-A and SAFE-C showing significant predictive ability. Adolescents who endorsed their American culture (higher VIA-A scores) reported lower social competence ratings. Further, higher acculturative stress (SAFE-C) scores predicted lower social competence ratings. The authors argue that their results were in line with developmental models of ethnic identity which posit that a strong ethnic identity is associated with better psychological well-being; however, this was not the case for social competence necessarily (Goforth et al., 2014).

Limitations of Goforth et al. (2014) included a small sample size that was obtained from a community containing a large number of Arab Americans. Further, Goforth et al. (2014) did not directly examine ethnic identity in their study and the association with overall mental health. The authors noted that this examination is important for future research because ethnic identity may provide a sense of collective support in facing discrimination and other acculturative stressors among Arab American adolescents. Finally, it should be noted that the perceived discrimination stress variable was not directly examined by itself in the regression models. This investigation may have been worthwhile in informing this relationship and should be considered in future research endeavors.

Conclusion

Arab cultures are severely misunderstood and portrayed negatively through the media in the United States. Consequently, Arabs in America face prejudice and discrimination from the mainstream public. These types of experiences have been found to impact self-concept and ethnic identity in various ethnic minority groups. The literature on adolescents of Arab descent in America has historically been limited but is more recently emerging. Nevertheless, results from the narrative review presented above are somewhat inconclusive. Only two studies were found that investigated self-concept and school environment, including discrimination. Both the studies found that discrimination was related to specific constructs of self-concept, particularly academic competence and physical appearance. Seven were found regarding ethnic identity and discrimination with varying results. In the qualitative studies, adolescents either pushed away from or pulled closer to their in-group peers in the face of discrimination. The quantitative studies reviewed either found no relationship or results contended with the rejection-identification model. Two studies were found that investigated psychological well-being in relation to discrimination, one qualitative and one quantitative. Both the studies showed evidence of a relationship between discrimination or perceived discrimination stress and mental health. Given the inconsistencies found across studies and the fact that there is a limited number of studies available, future studies are warranted to further investigate, confirm, and expand on these issues to inform researchers and practitioners on the various processes and factors related to developmental outcomes in adolescents of Arab descent in America.

References

Achenbach, T. M., & Rescorla, L. A. (2001). *Manual for the ASEBA school-age forms & profiles*. Burlington, VT: University of Vermont, Research Center for Children, Youth, and Families.

ADC. (2011). *The 2010 ADC legal report: Legal advocacy and policy review*. Washington, DC: American Arab Anti-Discrimination Committee.

Ahmed, S. R., Kia-Keating, M., & Tsai, K. H. (2011). A structural model of racial discrimination, acculturative stress, and cultural resources among Arab American adolescents. *American Journal of Community Psychology, 48*, 181–192. https://doi.org/10.1007/s10464-011-9424-3.

Albdour, M., Lewin, L., Kavanaugh, K., Hong, J. S., & Wilson, F. (2017). Arab American adolescents' perceived stress and bullying experiences: A qualitative study. *Western Journal of Nursing Research, 39*(12), 1567–1588. https://doi.org/10.1177/0193945916678214.

Al-Hazza, T., & Bucher, K. T. (2010). Bridging a cultural divide with literature about Arabs and Arab Americans. *Middle School Journal, 41*, 4–11. https://doi.org/10.2307/23047567.

Amer, M. M., & Kayyali, R. A. (2016). Religion and religiosity: Christian and Muslim faiths, diverse practices, and psychological correlates. In M. M. Amer & G. H. Awad (Eds.), *Handbook of Arab American psychology*. New York: Routledge.

Bayoumi, M. (2009). *How does it feel to be a problem?: Being young and Arab in America*. New York: Penguin.

Branscombe, N. R., Schmitt, M. T., & Harvey, R. D. (1999). Perceiving pervasive discrimination among African Americans: Implications for group identification and well-being. *Journal of Personality and Social Psychology, 77*(1), 135–149. https://doi.org/10.1037/0022-3514.77.1.135.

Cainkar, L. (2009). *Homeland insecurity: The Arab American and Muslim American experience after 9/11*. New York: Russell Sage Foundation.

Chavez, D. V., Moran, V. R., Reid, S. L., & Lopez, M. (1997). Acculturative stress in children: A modification of the SAFE scale. *Hispanic Journal of Behavioral Sciences, 19*(1), 34–44. https://doi.org/10.1177/07399863970191002.

Cohen, S., Kamarck, T., & Mermelstein, R. (1983). A global measure of perceived stress. *Journal of Health and Social Behavior, 24*(4), 385–396. https://doi.org/10.2307/2136404.

Crowne, D. P., & Marlowe, D. (1960). A new scale of social desirability independent of psychopathology. *Journal of Consulting Psychology, 24*(4), 349–354. https://doi.org/10.1037/h0047358.

Fiala, W. E., Bjorck, J. P., & Gorsuch, R. (2002). The religious support scale: Construction, validation, and cross-validation. *American Journal of Community Psychology, 30*(6), 761–786. https://doi.org/10.1023/A:1020264718397.

Finn, M., Hennebry, J., & Momani, B. (2018). Canadian Arab youth at the border: Cultural dissociation, fear management, and disciplining practices in securitized spaces. *Journal of International Migration and Integration, 19*(3), 667–682. https://doi.org/10.1007/s12134-018-0559-z.

Flanagan, C. A., Syvertsen, A. K., Gill, S., Gallay, L. S., & Cumsille, P. (2009). Ethnic awareness, prejudice, and civic commitments in four ethnic groups of American adolescents. *Journal of Youth and Adolescence, 38*(4), 19. https://doi.org/10.1007/s10964-009-9394-z.

Goforth, A. N., Oka, E. R., Leong, F. T. L., & Denis, D. J. (2014). Acculturation, acculturative stress, religiosity and psychological adjustment among Muslim Arab American adolescents. *Journal of Muslim Mental Health, 8*(2), 3–19. https://doi.org/10.3998/jmmh.10381607.0008.202.

Harter, S. (1985). *Manual for the self-perception profile for children*. Denver, CO: University of Denver.

Harter, S. (1988). *Manual for the self-perception profile for adolescents*. Denver, CO: University of Denver.

Ibish, H. E. (2001). *Report on hate crimes and discrimination against Arab Americans 1998–2000*. Washington, DC: American Arab Anti-Discrimination Committee Research Institute.

Kumar, R., Seay, N., & Karabenick, S. A. (2015). Immigrant Arab adolescents in ethnic enclaves: Physical and phenomenological contexts of identity negotiation. *Cultural Diversity and Ethnic Minority Psychology, 21*, 201–212. https://doi.org/10.1037/a0037748.

Kumar, R., Warnke, J. H., & Karabenick, S. A. (2014). Arab-American male identity negotiations: Caught in the crossroads of ethnicity, religion, nationality and current contexts. *Social Identities: Journal for the Study of Race, Nation and Culture, 20*(1), 22–41. https://doi.org/10.1080/13504630.2013.864464.

Najjar, K., Naser, S. C., & Clonan-Roy, K. (2019). Experiences of Arab heritage youth in US schools and impact on identity development. *School Psychology International., 40*, 251. https://doi.org/10.1177/0143034319831057.

Nyborg, V. M. (2000). I, too, sing America: Examining the racial experiences of African American boys and their relation to aggressive behavior. *Dissertation Abstracts International, 52*, 694.

Padilla, A. M., Wagatsuma, Y., & Lindholm, K. J. (1985). Acculturation and personality as predictors of stress in Japanese and Japanese-Americans. *The Journal of Social Psychology, 125*(3), 295–305. https://doi.org/10.1080/00224545.1985.9922890.

Pargament, K. I. (1999). *Multidimensional measurement of religiousness/spirituality for use in health research*. Retrieved April 28, 2019, from https://fetzer.org/resources/multidimensional-measurement-religiousnessspirituality-use-health-research

Pargament, K. I., Smith, B. W., Koenig, H. G., & Perez, L. (1998). Patterns of positive and negative religious coping with major life stressors. *Journal for the Scientific Study of Religion, 37*(4), 710–724. https://doi.org/10.2307/1388152.

Phinney, J. S. (1992). The multigroup ethnic identity measure: A new sclae for use with diverse groups. *Journal of Adolescent Research, 7*, 156–176.

Radloff, L. S. (1977). The CES-D scale: A self-report depression scale for research in the general population. *Applied Psychological Measurement, 1*(3), 385–401. https://doi.org/10.1177/014662167700100306.

Read, J. G. (2008). Discrimination and identity formation in post 9/11 era: A comparison of Muslim and Christian Arab Americans. In A. Jamal & N. Naber (Eds.), *Race and Arab Americans before and after 9/11: From invisible citizens to visible subjects* (pp. 305–317). Syracuse, NY: Syracuse University Press.

Ryder, A. G., Alden, L. E., & Paulhus, D. L. (2000). Is acculturation unidimensional or bidimensional? A head-to-head comparison in the prediction of personality, self-identity, and adjustment. *Journal of Personality and Social Psychology, 79*(1), 49–65. https://doi.org/10.1037//0022-3514.79.1.49.

Spielberger, C. D. (1983). *Manual for the state-trait anxiety inventory STAI (Form Y)*. Palo Alto, CA: Mind Garden.

Tabbah, R. (2021). Discrimination and developmental processes: Bridging the research gap with adolescents of Arab descent in America. *Adolescent Research Review, 6*(1), 1–13. https://doi.org/10.1007/s40894-019-00125-x.

Tabbah, R., Chung, J. J., & Miranda, A. H. (2016). Ethnic identity and discrimination: An exploration of the rejection-identification model in Arab American adolescents. *Identity, 16*(4), 319–334. https://doi.org/10.1080/15283488.2016.1231609.

Tabbah, R., Miranda, A. H., & Wheaton, J. E. (2012). Self-concept in Arab American adolescents: Implications of social support and experiences in the schools. *Psychology in the Schools, 49*, 817–827. https://doi.org/10.1002/pits.21640.

Tabbah, R., Miranda, A. H., & Wheaton, J. E. (2016). Intricacies of school relationships and the well-being of Arab American youth: Implications for school psychologists. *Contemporary School Psychology, 20*(4), 315–326. https://doi.org/10.1007/s40688-016-0089-7.

Tabbah, R., Wheaton, J. E., & Miranda, A. H. (2015). Finding identity without discrimination: The plight of Arab American adolescents. *Identities: Global Studies in Culture and Power, 23*, 519–535. https://doi.org/10.1080/1070289X.2015.1064423.

Wray-Lake, L., Syvertsen, A. K., & Flanagan, C. A. (2008). Contested citizenship and social exclusion: Adolescent Arab American immigrants' views of the social contract. *Applied Developmental Science, 12*, 84–92. https://doi.org/10.1080/10888690801997085.

Discrimination and Developmental Processes: Bridging the Research Gap on Arab American Youth

Introduction

The research on Arab American youth concerning discrimination and developmental processes is relatively scarce but more recently emerging since the terrorist attacks of 9/11. A review of existing studies reveals various methodological weaknesses and limitations, ranging from cross-sectional designs to recruitment difficulties to sampling issues. The purpose of this chapter is to identify the various limitations and gaps in the research on Arab American youth and provide strategies to address these issues. Given the relative lack of research available on Arab American youth, researchers need to increase and strengthen the body of evidence regarding these adolescents. This chapter provides guidance on how to reach this goal. The dialogue begins with an overview of the existing literature on Arab youth development and discrimination experiences. The overview focuses on methodological weaknesses found within each study. Then, common methodological weaknesses and limitations across studies are identified. Based on these findings, strategies are presented that researchers may implement to address these limitations, strengthen methodology, and increase the body of evidence available on Arab American youth and development outcomes related to their discrimination experiences.

An Overview of Existing Research on Arab Youth Development and Discrimination

A literature search regarding studies on Arab youth and discrimination in American revealed 11 studies. Two of these studies investigated various aspects of self-concept and discrimination in schools. Seven examined ethnic identity and two explored general well-being and psychological issues related to discrimination. This section

R. Tabbah, *Arab American Youth*, Advancing Responsible Adolescent Development, https://doi.org/10.1007/978-3-030-66804-4_8

provides an overview of these studies with a focus on methodological limitations found in each study and concludes with an identification of common weaknesses found across studies.

Two studies examined self-concept and discrimination in Arab American youth. First, Tabbah, Miranda, and Wheaton (2012) examined academic, social, and global aspects of self-concept in Arab American adolescents in relation to social supports and discrimination in the schools. Subsequently, Tabbah, Miranda, and Wheaton (2016) explored additional dimensions of self-concept—including physical appearance, athletic competence, behavioral conduct, and close friendship—with regard to social support and discrimination in the school system. These two studies utilized the same sample, procedures, and methodology. For both the studies, the authors implemented a cross-sectional design and utilized a purposive selection process as a result of having difficulty identifying and contacting Arab American adolescents to participate in the study. Therefore, they utilized snowball sampling to expedite the process, which limited generalizability. Related to this issue was the relatively small sample size, low response rates, and self-selection. Further limiting generalizability, most of the respondents resided in the Midwestern region of the United States. The authors noted that differences related to religious affiliation and generational status were not able to be examined due to small sample sizes. It was difficult to determine whether being of the Muslim faith was a contributing factor of discrimination experiences. Furthermore, in terms of generational status, second- and third-generation adolescents may have been less prone to discrimination than first-generation adolescents depending on their acculturation experiences. Finally, the nature of the discrimination questionnaire did not allow for the reporting of frequency of experiences and only focused on the school setting.

Seven studies were found examining the relationship between ethnic identity and discrimination with Arab American youth involving both community and school settings and using either qualitative or quantitative designs. Flanagan, Syvertsen, Gill, Gallay, and Cumsille (2009) examined the relationship between ethnic background, experiences of prejudice, and ethnic awareness with Arab American, African American, Latino American, and European American youth. The authors used a cross-sectional design and relied on self-report measures to collect data. The scales used on measures contained relatively few items, which likely affected the internal consistency of those measures. Furthermore, only one aspect of ethnic identity, ethnic awareness, was measured. Due to the cross-sectional nature, the authors were not able to examine changes in ethnic awareness and identity over time and in response to experiences in different contexts.

Kumar, Warnke, and Karabenick (2014) focused on identity in Arab American male adolescents in the Midwestern region of the United States relative to public perception, experiences of discrimination, and stereotype awareness. The authors utilized a cross-sectional design and qualitative measures through focus-group interviews. Participants were randomly selected from a single community. The cross-sectional nature limited any detection of changes in identity over time and related to different social adversities and political conditions. While the randomized selection of participants was a strength, selection from one community limited generalization.

Kumar, Seay, and Karabenick (2015) conducted a cross-sectional, qualitative study examining identity negotiations of recent Arab immigrants who were randomly selected. Similar to the previous study, randomized selection of participants was a strength. However, the focus-group nature and the selection of participants from one community limited generalizability. Additionally, the cross-sectional nature limited any detection of changes in identity over time and related to different social adversities and political conditions.

Next, Tabbah, Wheaton, and Miranda (2015) examined the aspects of ethnic identity and discrimination experiences in the school system. The authors utilized snowball sampling, a cross-sectional design, and a relatively small sample size. The study sample was not considered representative of the Arab American population, as the sample majority was Muslim and the Arab American population majority is actually Christian (Amer & Kayyali, 2016). The authors also reported difficulty in the selection process due to complications with identifying Arab American participants. Therefore, the sample had to be selected purposively, which also limited the generalizability of the results. Important factors such as generational status were not taken into consideration due to small group sizes.

Ahmed, Kia-Keating, and Tsai (2011) investigated racial discrimination, acculturative stress, and ethnic identity in relation to psychological distress in Arab American adolescents. The researchers utilized a cross-sectional design, which prevented the authors from measuring causal directionality of cultural resources and socio-cultural adversities on psychological distress. Further, students were self-selected for participation and the authors suggested that students who experienced more adversities may have been more prone to participating in the study. Generalizability was also limited due to the sampling taking place in a single community and also due to the sample being primarily Muslim. The latter does not allow reflection on the experiences of Arab Christian counterparts.

Tabbah, Chung, and Miranda (2016) investigated the aspects of ethnic identity, academic and global self-concept, and discrimination in the school system. The researchers utilized a cross-sectional design, relatively small sample size, and the use of purposive selection with the use of volunteers due to difficulties identifying Arab American participants. As a result of small sample size, the authors reported difficulty accounting for important variables in their results. While generational status was taken into consideration, the sample sizes may have been too small to detect any true differences. Also, due to small sample sizes, differences in Arab nationality were not able to be examined. The study sample was not considered representative of the Arab American population regarding nationality and religious affiliation, as the sample majority was Muslim and the Arab American population majority is Christian. These issues along with purposive sampling limited the generalizability of the results.

Najjar, Naser, and Clonan-Roy (2019) conducted a qualitative focus-group study with Arab American early college students and community dwellers where participants were asked to reflect on their primary school experiences with discrimination and how this related to their identity development. Najjar et al. (2019) was a cross-sectional study that utilized snowball sampling within one university and geographic region within the United States. Also, the study involved collecting retroactive data from individuals who had graduated from high school and were either currently involved in undergraduate studies or had earned a bachelor's degree.

In terms of general well-being and discrimination, only two studies were found, one related to school experiences and one to community experiences. First, Albdour, Lewin, Kavanaugh, Hong, and Wilson (2017) conducted a qualitative study that examined bullying experiences related to stress and anxiety in Arab American youth. The majority of these experiences were related to their race/ethnicity. Albdour et al. (2017) was a cross-sectional study including a small number of participants from one geographical area. In addition, the results relied on self-report with no confirmation from other sources, which the authors note may have increased the credibility of their findings. Finally, the authors did not account for other influential factors of stress that may have affected their findings (Albdour et al., 2017).

Second, Goforth, Oka, Leong, and Denis (2014) examined acculturation, acculturative stress, religiosity, and psychological adjustment in Muslim Arab American adolescents. Acculturative stress involved measures of perceived discrimination stress. This cross-sectional study utilized a small convenience sample that was obtained from a community containing a large number of Arab Americans. The sample consisted of all Muslim participants. Further, the authors did not directly examine ethnic identity in their study and the association with overall mental health. They noted that this examination is important for future research because ethnic identity may provide a sense of collective support in facing discrimination and other acculturative stressors among Arab American adolescents. Finally, it should be noted that the perceived discrimination stress variable was not directly examined by itself in regression analyses. This investigation may have been worthwhile in informing the relationship between perceived discrimination stress, acculturation statues, and psychological adjustment. Therefore, future research may consider examining this relationship.

An examination of the limitations across the studies presented above reveals several common issues. All studies were cross-sectional in nature. With the exception of Kumar et al.'s studies, all studies utilized convenience sampling. Even though Kumar and colleagues utilized random sampling in their method, the sample was chosen from one location, which then limits generalizability to that location. That being said, recruitment challenges exist because of the racial classification system for Arabs in the United States, which complicates sampling methods for researchers. Further limitations include the addition of study variables to be considered that may serve as confounding or influential factors. Finally, a common issue found regarded the use of psychometric measures that were not normed for Arab populations. The following sections outline these limitations and focus on strategies to address these issues in order to increase and strengthen the evidence regarding Arab American youth.

Methodology: Cross-Sectionality, Convenience Sampling, Racial Classification, and Recruitment Challenges

The existing literature presented consisted of a number of pilot studies that were mainly exploratory in nature and require replication with more rigorous methods, including sampling procedures and recruiting larger and more diverse samples. All of the research found regarding this group utilized cross-sectional designs, in which the data represented only one time point. Therefore, changes in developmental processes over time and in relation to different experiences could not be examined in any of the studies. Future research needs to take a longitudinal approach, in order to determine causal directionality of discrimination on these developmental processes.

Convenience sampling was another limitation to all studies with the exception of Kumar et al. (2014) and Kumar et al. (2015), where random sampling was used within one community. Although this strategy maximizes engagement at the community level, convenience sampling limits the generalizability of the results at hand (Shara et al., 2016). Often, Arab Americans may be distrustful of researchers and reluctant to participate in studies (Jaber, 2003), especially with the negative sociopolitical effects post-9/11 (Amer & Hovey, 2005). Therefore, convenience sampling allows for researchers to build more trust and connection through community leaders and focus on the visibility and accessibility of a particular study in locations that are regularly visited by the target study population (Shara et al., 2016). This method, combined with the building of trusting relationships, also improves retention rates in studies on this population relative to more random and systematic sampling methods used where this type of relationship building may not be realistic or practical (Shara et al., 2016).

Related to convenience sampling, many of the authors noted problems with selection due to difficulties identifying Arab participants in America. This problem stems from the limitations of racial classification systems in the United States that typically categorizes Arabs as white (Awad, Kia-Keating, & Amer, 2019). While random sampling is the best method for obtaining a representative sample, the racial classification system makes it almost impossible to readily identify this population. Researchers should be aware that the Arab American Institute (AAI) is actively working on this issue to add Arab ancestry on to the United States Census. Until then, researchers will have to continue to reach out to Arab American organizations to help with advertisement and recruiting participants or actively work on finding ways to identify this population. That being said, areas containing Arab American organizations are usually largely populated with Arabs. Consequently, Arabs living as a minority in other regions of the country are left out of these research opportunities. Further limiting generalizability of the studies cited, most of the studies chose participants from one region of the United States. Future studies should endeavor to reach multiple regions, in order to increase representation and generalizability. The largest populations live in California, Michigan, New York, Florida, Texas, New Jersey, Illinois, Ohio, Pennsylvania, and Virginia (AAI, n.d.). While some studies specified that they took place in ethnic enclaves, most studies cited did not specify this, and therefore, it is not known whether participants' experiences took place within or outside of such communities. Future research should consider comparing the experiences of participants living inside and outside of ethnic enclaves.

In addition to region, the religious diversity obtained for these studies was limited with largely Muslim samples, whereas the Arab American population is largely Christian (Amer & Kayyali, 2016). Future research should include larger samples of Arab Christians to investigate their experiences and perhaps compare their experiences to those of Arab Muslims. For example, one study compared discrimination experiences and psychological distress in Christian Arab American and Muslim Arab American adults (Abdulrahim, James, Yamout, & Baker, 2012). The authors found that discrimination was more frequently reported by Muslim Arab Americans, those who racially identified as non-white, and who lived in ethnic enclaves. However, the relationship between discrimination and psychological distress was stronger for Christian Arab Americans, those who racially identified as white, who have dark skin color, and who live outside of ethnic enclaves. Examining these same processes comparatively with Christian and Muslim Arab adolescents is worthwhile for future research and will provide a voice to represent the Christian population. Related to religion, the use of samples consisting primarily of Muslim participants may have served as a confounding factor in most of the studies cited in this narrative review, as it is difficult to determine the relative contribution of discrimination toward being of Muslim faith versus being a non-Muslim since there was a minimal sample of non-Muslims to compare (Tabbah, Chung, & Miranda, 2016).

Two studies were found that addressed recruitment challenges for Arab populations and implemented various strategies to determine their effectiveness in obtaining Arab samples. Kayrouz, Dear, Karin, and Titov (2016) proposed the use of Facebook as an effective recruitment strategy for hard-to-reach populations, specifically Arab populations. While their study was conducted in Australia, they used Facebook to recruit Arab participants worldwide for an Internet-based treatment for depression and anxiety. The larger study aimed to evaluate the efficacy and acceptability of a culturally modified version of an evidence-based treatment, the Wellbeing Course, for use with Arab individuals (Kayrouz et al., 2016). They compared recruitment through Facebook to traditional recruitment.

Traditional recruitment strategies were active for 14 weeks and involved a media release by the university media and communications department to relevant media organizations; emails with attached flyers to 94 different relevant Arab organizations, 108 health professionals, and approximately 80 interested individuals; two newspaper advertisements in English and two editorials in Arabic in an Australian Arabic newspaper; flyers in English in religious organizations and the Australian Lebanese Medical Association's newsletter; and information about the research on websites of the university and five mental health-related organizations (Kayrouz et al., 2016). The authors resorted to Facebook recruitment strategies after experiencing a slow rate of recruitment from these traditional strategies.

The Facebook strategy was implemented for 28 weeks and involved the creation of a personal profile and a dedicated Facebook public fan page about the research. Four promotion strategies were implemented: promoting posts regarding the research through boosting, promoting the Facebook public fan page for the research project, promoting websites for the research project, and promoting events through the personal profile and public fan page by inviting friends to participate in a research event. A total of 81 participants were recruited for the final sample through a combination of traditional and Facebook recruitment strategies.

While using Facebook was not more cost-effective, the use of this strategy served to be more effective in recruiting a study sample of Arab participants. The researchers were able to recruit only 11 participants through traditional recruitment strategies over the course of 42 weeks, whereas they were able to obtain an additional 70 participants through Facebook strategies. Kayrouz et al. (2016) cited the use of Facebook to recruit hard-to-reach populations as an effective strategy in combination with traditional measures. One downfall to Internet-based sampling methods, however, is the bias they likely hold toward younger populations who are more technologically savvy and participants who are richer and/or more educated (Clay, 2011).

Another study addressing recruitment challenges utilized a strategy called the "cycle-of-trust framework," which suggests using culturally sensitive methods during four stages, in order to enhance recruitment and retention: prior to study initiation, during recruitment, throughout the duration of the study, and after study completion (Shara et al., 2016, p. 33). Shara et al. (2016) urged the importance of utilizing community leaders and educators in building trust with potential research participants. These key stakeholders can play a major role in engaging community members in research studies by assuring participants that the research is beneficial and that it can be conducted in a culturally sensitive manner by emphasizing privacy and confidentiality (Shara et al., 2016).

Moreover, the use of culturally appropriate methods for conducting studies specifically with Arab populations is critical. In preparation for their study, Shara et al. (2016) searched the literature for appropriate strategies to use with this population. Also, one of their Arab American researchers trained the remaining research staff in culturally appropriate approaches, specifically issues related to Muslim women and their possible preference to being interviewed by a female researcher and/or being seen privately rather than in front of others (Shara et al., 2016).

Consideration of Additional Study Variables

Attaining a strong ethnic identity is important developmentally. However, exposure to various forms of discrimination may prevent adolescents from developing a healthy sense of acculturation and may cause them to have difficulty integrating with society (Hakim-Larson & Menna, 2016). A healthy acculturation process may lead to healthy self-concept, strong health, and a clear sense of identity (Najjar et al., 2019), while a maladaptive acculturative process may lead to a higher risk of psychological disorders and identity confusion (Amer & Hovey, 2007). Therefore, further examination of acculturation and acculturative stress related to discrimination and ethnic identity is warranted. While Ahmed et al. (2011) found that acculturative stress and discrimination were associated, there was no moderation of ethnic identity found on the effects of acculturative stress on psychological distress. Research with other ethnic minorities has shown that high levels of perceived discrimination attenuated negative associations between acculturation and ethnic identity (Baldwin-White, Kiehne, Umaña-Taylor, & Marsiglia, 2017). More research is needed to determine how such experiences affect this process in adolescents of Arab descent in America. Future researchers may consider testing various theoretical models to determine specific processes that are relevant to this adolescent group. It particularly would be important to include later generations and compare to first-generation adolescents as they may have highly different experiences.

The existing literature has provided evidence that the school climate is associated with the developmental processes of self-concept and ethnic identity in adolescents of Arab descent in America. In particular, teacher and peer support and interactions, discrimination experiences, and cultural representation and allowance of cultural expression in the schools were found to be important in the development of these adolescents. Consequently, future research endeavors need to address school climate in addition to community experiences. Najjar et al. (2019) would be particularly important to replicate with students currently attending school, perhaps using a mixed methods approach to gather both quantitative and qualitative measures.

Norming Psychometric Measures and Assessments for Arab Populations

Finally, most of the psychometric measures used in these studies were not necessarily normed with Arab populations in America. For example, Ahmed et al. (2011) changed the wording in their measures to match the ethnicity and religious affiliations of their participants; while their alphas obtained for each measure for the study sample were high, this might not be the case for future studies. Therefore, future research on measure development should consider including Arab descent populations in their normative samples. Two studies were found that attempted to validate translated scales for Arab populations in Lebanon and Saudi Arabia. Mahfoud et al. (2011) examined the—then recently developed—Arab Youth Mental Health scale as a screening measure for depression/anxiety in a sample of 153 Lebanese youth between the ages of 10 and 14 years. While results showed good internal consistency and specificity, the scale showed only moderate sensitivity for girls and poor sensitivity for boys. Therefore, the authors concluded that the scale was appropriate for the screening of depression and anxiety in girls of Arab culture but not necessarily for boys. Darraj et al. (2016) sought to validate an Arabic version of the Depression Literacy Questionnaire among an adolescent sample of 120 from four intermediate and secondary schools in a city in Saudi Arabia. The authors translated the items of the Depression Literacy Questionnaire into Arabic and administered it to the participants. Results regarding internal consistency and validity of the Arabic version were consistent with the English version of the measure showing solid support for its use with adolescent school students. Results from the factor analysis provided further support to construct validity of the Arabic version of the measure as all items were explained by a single factor indicating that it is a valid measure of depression literacy. Studies similar to the ones discussed above should be replicated with other measures, in order to determine their suitability with Arab American populations.

Conclusion

A review of the literature reveals various methodological weaknesses within studies available on Arab American youth. The limited number of studies currently available regarding Arab American youth experiences and developmental outcomes, along with the inconsistencies and limitations found across and within results and methodology, calls for future research to validate and strengthen the evidence available. Common limitations found across studies included sampling procedures, recruitment difficulties, cross-sectional designs, examination of additional variables, and lack of measures normed on Arab populations. The majority of studies utilized convenience sampling or sampled randomly from one location, both which limit generalizability of results. Furthermore, most studies utilized samples that consisted primarily of Muslim participants, which does not allow for the examination of various religions to see if experiences differ. Related to sampling procedures, recruitment difficulties were cited by many authors. Due to Arabs being racially classified as white, researchers have difficulty identifying Arabs for recruitment. All studies were cross-sectional, which does not allow for the examination of cause and effect and changes in development across time. Additionally, researchers may consider additional variables in their studies that play an important role in development, such as acculturation and/or acculturation stress. Finally, psychometric measures that have been normed with Arabs are lacking, leaving researchers with the need to adapt existing measures, which may influence validity. Therefore, future research may focus on the development and validation of measures for Arab American youth. This chapter focused on various strategies that researchers may consider to address these issues when conducting future research with this population.

References

AAI. (n.d.). *Demographics*. Retrieved September 23, 2019, from http://www.aaiusa.org/demographics

Abdulrahim, S., James, S. A., Yamout, R., & Baker, W. (2012). Discrimination and psychological distress: Does whiteness matter for Arab Americans? *Social Science & Medicine, 75*(12), 2116–2123. https://doi.org/10.1016/j.socscimed.2012.07.030.

Ahmed, S. R., Kia-Keating, M., & Tsai, K. H. (2011). A structural model of racial discrimination, acculturative stress, and cultural resources among Arab American adolescents. *American Journal of Community Psychology, 48*, 181–192. https://doi.org/10.1007/s10464-011-9424-3.

Albdour, M., Lewin, L., Kavanaugh, K., Hong, J. S., & Wilson, F. (2017). Arab American adolescents' perceived stress and bullying experiences: A qualitative study. *Western Journal of Nursing Research, 39*(12), 1567–1588. https://doi.org/10.1177/0193945916678214.

Amer, M. M., & Hovey, J. D. (2005). Examination of the impact of acculturation, stress, and religiosity on mental health variables for second-generation Arab Americans. *Ethnicity and Disease, 15*, S1-111–S1-112.

Amer, M. M., & Hovey, J. D. (2007). Socio-demographic differences in acculturation and mental health for a sample of 2nd generation/early immigrant Arab Americans. *Journal of Immigrant and Minority Health, 9*, 335. https://doi.org/10.1007/s10903-007-9045-y.

Amer, M. M., & Kayyali, R. A. (2016). Religion and religiosity: Christian and Muslim faiths, diverse practices, and psychological correlates. In M. M. Amer & G. H. Awad (Eds.), *Handbook of Arab American psychology*. New York: Routledge.

Awad, G. H., Kia-Keating, M., & Amer, M. M. (2019). A model of cumulative racial–ethnic trauma among Americans of Middle Eastern and North African (MENA) descent. *American Psychologist, 74*(1), 76–87. https://doi.org/10.1037/amp0000344.

Baldwin-White, A. J. M., Kiehne, E., Umaña-Taylor, A., & Marsiglia, F. F. (2017). Pursuit of belonging: Acculturation, perceived discrimination, and ethnic-racial identity among Latino youths. *Social Work Research, 41*(1), 43–52. https://doi.org/10.1093/swr/svw029.

Clay, R. A. (2011). Muslims in America, post 9/11. *Monitor on Psychology, 42*(8). Retrieved from http://www.apa.org/monitor/2011/09/muslims

Darraj, H. A., Mahfouz, M. S., Al Sanosi, R. M., Badedi, M., Sabai, A., Al Refaei, A., et al. (2016). Arabic translation and psychometric evaluation of the Depression Literacy Questionnaire among adolescents. *Psychiatry Journal, 2016*, 8045262. https://doi.org/10.1155/2016/8045262.

Flanagan, C. A., Syvertsen, A. K., Gill, S., Gallay, L. S., & Cumsille, P. (2009). Ethnic awareness, prejudice, and civic commitments in four ethnic groups of American adolescents. *Journal of Youth and Adolescence, 38*(4), 19. https://doi.org/10.1007/s10964-009-9394-z.

Goforth, A. N., Oka, E. R., Leong, F. T. L., & Denis, D. J. (2014). Acculturation, acculturative stress, religiosity and psychological adjustment among Muslim Arab American adolescents. *Journal of Muslim Mental Health, 8*(2), 3–19. https://doi.org/10.3998/jmmh.10381607.0008.202.

Hakim-Larson, J., & Menna, R. (2016). Acculturation and enculturation: Ethnic identity socialization process. In M. M. Amer & G. H. Awad (Eds.), *Handbook of Arab American psychology* (pp. 34–47). New York: Routledge.

Jaber, L. A. (2003). Barriers and strategies for research in Arab Americans. *Diabetes Care, 26*(2), 514–515. https://doi.org/10.2337/diacare.26.2.514.

Kayrouz, R., Dear, B. F., Karin, E., & Titov, N. (2016). Facebook as an effective recruitment strategy for mental health research of hard to reach populations. *Internet Interventions, 4*, 1–10. https://doi.org/10.1016/j.invent.2016.01.001.

Kumar, R., Seay, N., & Karabenick, S. A. (2015). Immigrant Arab adolescents in ethnic enclaves: Physical and phenomenological contexts of identity negotiation. *Cultural Diversity and Ethnic Minority Psychology, 21*, 201–212. https://doi.org/10.1037/a0037748.

Kumar, R., Warnke, J. H., & Karabenick, S. A. (2014). Arab-American male identity negotiations: Caught in the crossroads of ethnicity, religion, nationality and current contexts. *Social Identities: Journal for the Study of Race, Nation and Culture, 20*(1), 22–41. https://doi.org/10.1080/13504630.2013.864464.

Mahfoud, Z., Abdulrahim, S., Taha, M. B., Harpham, T., El Hajj, T., Makhoul, J., et al. (2011). Validation of the Arab Youth Mental Health scale as a screening tool for depression/anxiety in

Lebanese children. *Child and Adolescent Psychiatry and Mental Health, 5*, 9–9. https://doi.org/10.1186/1753-2000-5-9.

Najjar, K., Naser, S. C., & Clonan-Roy, K. (2019). Experiences of Arab heritage youth in US schools and impact on identity development. *School Psychology International, 40*, 251. https://doi.org/10.1177/0143034319831057.

Shara, N. M., Yassin, S., Abu-Bader, S. H., Getaneh, A., Browning, S. M., Zeymo, A., et al. (2016). Overcoming recruitment challenges: A pilot study in Arab Americans. *Journal of Health Disparities Research and Practice, 9*, 3. Retrieved from https://digitalscholarship.unlv.edu/cgi/viewcontent.cgi?article=1427&context=jhdrp

Tabbah, R., Chung, J. J., & Miranda, A. H. (2016). Ethnic identity and discrimination: An exploration of the rejection-identification model in Arab American adolescents. *Identity, 16*(4), 319–334. https://doi.org/10.1080/15283488.2016.1231609.

Tabbah, R., Miranda, A. H., & Wheaton, J. E. (2012). Self-concept in Arab American adolescents: Implications of social support and experiences in the schools. *Psychology in the Schools, 49*, 817–827. https://doi.org/10.1002/pits.21640.

Tabbah, R., Miranda, A. H., & Wheaton, J. E. (2016). Intricacies of school relationships and the Well-being of Arab American youth: Implications for school psychologists. *Contemporary School Psychology, 20*(4), 315–326. https://doi.org/10.1007/s40688-016-0089-7.

Tabbah, R., Wheaton, J. E., & Miranda, A. H. (2015). Finding identity without discrimination: The plight of Arab American adolescents. *Identities: Global Studies in Culture and Power, 23*, 519–535. https://doi.org/10.1080/1070289X.2015.1064423.

Transforming Education Practice and Policy for Arab American Youth

Introduction

Research regarding Arab American youth and their developmental outcomes related to their experiences in the school system is limited. Nevertheless, results consistently demonstrate a significant negative relation between school discrimination experiences and various aspects of development. Therefore, we may begin to imply that there is an impact of discrimination experiences on developmental processes in Arab American adolescents. Although the research is scarce, the preliminary evidence may be used to inform policy and practice in the K-12 school system for Arab American students.

The purpose of this chapter is to present the areas of educational practice and policy that need to be addressed to effectively serve Arab American youth. The chapter offers strategies relevant in the reform of these areas. Due to perpetual cultural misconceptions, it is critical for policy to focus on multicultural reform in the education system, in order to more thoroughly and accurately represent Arab and Arab American cultures. School practitioners and educators need to be informed of school climate, its effects on students, and strategies that may improve the environment to better serve this adolescent population.

This chapter begins with an overview of the research on Arab American youth regarding discrimination in school systems. The discussion focuses on identifying common themes across studies related to the various levels and factors of the school environment that need to be addressed. Identified areas include cultural awareness at all school levels, staff development of cultural competence, peer and teacher relationships—especially intercultural relationships among peers—and curriculum reform. The chapter discusses each of these areas in detail. To address cultural awareness and competence, first, there is a presentation of general common factors of Arab American cultures to help educators build some cultural awareness and knowledge. Then, the journey to cultural competence for educators regarding Arab American youth is described. The next area addressed involves peer and teacher

R. Tabbah, *Arab American Youth*, Advancing Responsible Adolescent Development, https://doi.org/10.1007/978-3-030-66804-4_9

relations with a focus on building intercultural relationships. A thorough discussion on various strategies to implement in order to build and improve intercultural relations in schools is provided. This is followed by the final area identified, which is curricula. Strategies and methods for reforming curricula to include and accurately represent Arab cultures are presented. Given that the research provides evidence that school discrimination experiences is related to various developmental factors, the chapter concludes with a dialogue regarding intervention strategies relevant to Arab American students in terms of development with a focus on mental health.

An Overview of Research on School Experiences and Developmental Outcomes in Arab Youth

A literature search revealed 11 studies examining discrimination experiences and developmental outcomes in Arab American youth. Eight of these studies included examination of discrimination experiences in school (Albdour, Lewin, Kavanaugh, Hong, & Wilson, 2017; Kumar, Seay, & Karabenick, 2015; Kumar, Warnke, & Karabenick, 2014; Najjar, Naser, & Clonan-Roy, 2019; Tabbah, Chung, & Miranda, 2016; Tabbah, Miranda, & Wheaton, 2012, 2016; Tabbah, Wheaton, & Miranda, 2015). That being said, four of these studies (Tabbah et al., 2012, 2015; Tabbah, Chung, & Miranda, 2016; Tabbah, Miranda, & Wheaton, 2016) used the same sample across studies, leaving us with five unique investigations of school experiences. In all studies reviewed, results indicate that the school environment influences various aspects of development in Arab American adolescents.

In summary, Albdour et al. (2017) found that bullying experiences in Arab American youth were associated with high levels of stress and anxiety. The majority of these experiences were related to their race/ethnicity. In a retrospective study by Najjar et al. (2019), school factors influencing identity negotiations in a sample of Arab American adolescents included peer and teacher discrimination, the treatment of Arab history and culture in the school curriculum, and the allowance for student cultural expression through broader school structures. School discrimination was found to be significantly, negatively related to classmate support and academic (Tabbah et al., 2012) and physical appearance (Tabbah, Miranda, & Wheaton, 2016) aspects of self-concept. In another study, Tabbah et al. (2015) indicated that school discrimination was positively related to aspects of ethnic identity, in line with the rejection-identification model. The authors found that ethnic identity search was significantly, positively related to both discrimination of self and discrimination of others. Affirmation/belonging was positively related to discrimination of self only. Further, the multiple experiences group held the highest means on both ethnic identity search and affirmation/belonging subscales. Those in the multiple experiences group had significantly higher mean scores than those in the no discrimination group on both ethnic identity search and affirmation/belonging measures.

In a subsequent investigation, Tabbah, Chung, and Miranda (2016) revealed that discrimination and aspects of ethnic identity were significantly associated with factors of self-concept. To reiterate, the authors found that discrimination and lower affirmation/belonging of ethnic identity significantly predicted lower levels of academic self-concept. While discrimination was not related to global self-worth, higher levels of affirmation/belonging predicted higher levels of global self-worth.

In a sample of male Arab American adolescents, Kumar et al. (2014) found that their devalued status in society reinforced their identities and, in the face of social and political adversities, reinforced a need to be surrounded by their in-group members. Their identity negotiations were complicated further by being born and growing up in the post-9/11 era. Students in the sample who attended a predominantly white school reported feeling disenfranchised. Their personal and group experiences were not valued by their peers and teachers. The authors indicated that these experiences may lead to a stronger identification with their in-group and distrust of outgroup members. The authors also reported that the salience of social identities depended on the cultural diversity within the school framework. For example, students who attended the more culturally diverse schools were required to confront and negotiate the meaning of their social identities within their own groups and their perceptions of intergroup relations in school. The authors found greater intragroup variability in the identity negotiations of students attending these schools. The authors reported evidence that in schools where intergroup and intercultural contact was common, participants' self-identification ranged on the assimilation continuum from desire to assimilate as an American to a strong Arab identity that denounced American status. On the contrary, students attending predominantly Arab/Arab American schools with less intercultural contact stated more comfort and a strong sense of belonging to the school and the Muslim and/or Arab American community. These students did not have to battle with the daily exposure to discrimination or prejudice. The authors concluded that, for these adolescents, the school and community buffered against societal stereotyping, prejudice, and discrimination. In addition, these adolescents identified themselves based on the country of origin in order to preserve optimal distinctiveness.

In Kumar et al. (2015), identity negotiations of recent Arab immigrants were influenced by whether or not their school was located within an ethnic enclave and by the cultural competencies of school staff. Specifically, recent immigrants attending schools within ethnic enclaves felt a sense of comfort from having their cultural and religious values reflected in the environment. Further, school staff within schools of ethnic enclaves were deemed more culturally competent in their practice with students. That being said, within ethnic enclave schools, immigrant students reported a hierarchical status of Arab students based on nationality and were bullied depending on their nationality/country of origin by other Arab students. Bullying and taunting consisted of name-calling, discrimination, and rejection. Students sometimes felt invalidated by their teachers and peers, who would challenge the meaning and value of immigrants' cultural and religious identity. Staff ignored their reports when these students' sought help. Finally, conflict and confusion were created for both male and female participants due to misunderstanding and perceived misinterpretation of their behaviors by teachers. The authors speculated that these reactions may have been fueled by teachers' biased views mirroring societal negative stereotypes and prejudices of the Arab community.

Results from these studies inform on the various aspects of the school environment as well as educational policies that continue to need reform. Areas that need to be addressed include cultural awareness, school staff development of cultural competence, peer and teacher relationships, including intercultural relationships among peers, curriculum representation, and school policies regarding culture. The remainder of this chapter focuses on these issues. First, because of the importance of understanding a culture to develop cultural competence, a more detailed discussion regarding the various aspects of Arab American cultures is presented.

Important Factors of Arab American Cultures

Various resources and articles are available to learn about Arab cultures (e.g., Goforth, Nichols, Stanick, Shindorf, & Holter, 2017; Haboush, 2007; Hakim-Larson, Kamoo, Nassar-McMillan, & Porcerelli, 2007; Wingfield, 2006). Table 1, originally from Goforth et al. (2017), displays some excellent references for school staff to utilize in their journey of learning about Arab cultures. Haboush (2007) provided an excellent overview of Arab cultures as general guidelines for school psychologists working with Arab American families. However, these guidelines may be considered relevant for all school staff. The author emphasized that these points are considered general guidelines only, since variability exists among all Arab families (Haboush, 2007). While there are indeed commonalities, not every Arab American family necessarily holds each of these characteristics. Therefore, it is crucial for school staff to specifically learn about the various values and characteristics each of their students and their families embrace. Each family is going to have different experiences depending on their immigration history, country of origin, religion, and family values. Therefore, it is crucial for staff working with Arab families to be aware of these differences that may influence development of relationships with each family. Haboush (2007) covered central aspects of Arab culture, such as areas of demographics, perceptions of education, perceptions of mental health, religion, and family. For effective practice purposes in building rapport, researchers suggest that school staff working with Arab American families show interest in learning about their cultural traditions and religion (Erickson & Al-Timimi, 2001). It is also imperative to understand the history of colonization, as well as their immigration experiences, and the potential effects these have had on the Arab psyche.

Table 1 Resources and materials related to Arab Americans (Goforth et al., 2017)

Topic	Resource	Citation or link	Brief description
Arab American history, religion, and culture	Arab American Institute (AAI)	www.aaiusa.org	AAI is a non-profit leadership organization dedicated to representing the community interests of Arabs in America. Information on Arab American demographics, education, and statistics is provided
	The American Arab National Museum (AANM)	www.arabamericanmuseum.org	The AANM is the first and only museum to dedicate itself to the history and culture of Arab Americans. Information and publications are available on Arab American history and culture
	The American-Arab Anti-Discrimination Committee	www.adc.org/education/educational-resources/	Largest Arab American civil rights of the people of Arab descent. Free downloadable resources and lesson plans are available that addresses a variety of topics from examining Arab stereotypes, facts about Islam, and Arab American history
	Handbook of Arab American psychology	Amer, M.M. & Awad, G.H. (Eds.). (2016). Handbook of Arab American psychology. New York, NY: Routledge	Edited book that provides a comprehensive overview of psychological research related to Arab Americans
Counseling and interventions	*Counseling the culturally diverse: theory and practice*	Sue, D.W. & Sue, D. (2013) Counseling the culturally diverse: theory and practice. Hoboken, NJ: John Wiley & Sons	Provides text on understanding culturally diverse clients with one chapter specific to counseling Arab and Muslim Americans
	Counseling and Diversity: Counseling Arab Americans	Nassar-McMillan, S., Choudhuri, D.D., & Santiago-Rivera, A. (2010). Counseling & diversity: counseling Arab Americans	Resource to understand how to provide culturally responsive counseling to Arab Americans
	Counseling considerations among Arab Americans	Nassar-McMillan, S.C. & Hakim-Larson, J. (2003). Counseling considerations among Arab Americans. Journal of Counseling & Development, 81, 150–159	Review of best practices for counseling Arab Americans
	Considerations for school psychologists working with Arab American children and families	Goforth, A.N. (2011). Considerations for school psychologists working with Arab American children and families. Communique, 39, 28–30	Review of best practices for school psychological services (assessment and intervention)
	Key issues to consider in therapy with Muslim families	Weatherhead, S., & Daiches, A. (2015). Key issues to consider in therapy with Muslim families. Journal of Religion and Health, 54, 2398–2411	Clinical implications of culture and Islam when providing therapy to Muslim families

(continued)

Table 1 (continued)

Topic	Resource	Citation or link	Brief description
Assessment of diverse youth	*Assessing Culturally and Linguistically Diverse Students: A Practice Guide*	Rhodes, R.L., Ochoa, S.H., & Ortiz, S.O. (2005). Assessing culturally and linguistically diverse students: a practical guide. New York: Guilford Press	A practical guide to the process of non-discriminatory assessment
	RTI network: considerations for English Language Learners	http://rtinetwork.org/getstarted/sld-identification-toolkit/ld-identification-toolkit-considerations-for-ell	Practical overview of how to assess English language learners at multi-tiered systems of support
Refugees	U.S. Committee for Refugees and Immigrants	www.refugees.org/resources	Resource library and resources for refugees, immigrants, and people who support them
	Office of Refugee Resettlement, Department of Health and Human Services	www.acf.hhs.gov/programs/orr/refugees	Information relevant for refugees, including social services and programs, health services, and resettlement programs

Reprinted by permission from Springer Nature Customer Service Centre GmbH: Springer Nature *Contemporary School Psychology* School-Based Considerations for Supporting Arab American Youths' Mental Health, Anisa N. Goforth et al., ©2016

Demographics

Arabs are defined by the United States Census Bureau as those whose ancestry originated in any of the Arabic-speaking countries, although not all individuals in these countries necessarily consider themselves to be Arabs (i.e., Kurds and Berbers) (de la Cruz & Brittingham, 2003). There are 22 Arab countries across the Middle East and North Africa that all differ in racial and ethnic mix, religious composition, and economic development (Haboush, 2007). Racial diversity is not reflected accurately in the United States Census because they are officially considered white by the government (Haboush, 2007).

Haboush (2007) cited several disputes throughout history regarding religion, territorial boundaries, and political dominance that have influenced Arab culture. During the Crusades, many Arab countries were taken over by various foreign powers including the Ottomans, English, French, and Italians. European colonization combined with the devaluation of Arab cultures that was endured well into the mid-twentieth century contributed to feelings of mistrust toward the West (Erickson & Al-Timimi, 2001). In addition, the Crusades led to a divide between Christian and Muslim groups who view each other as a threat (e.g., Lebanese Civil War; Haboush, 2007). Moreover, internal divisions exist within each of these groups, for example, Sunni and Shiite sects of Islam (Haboush, 2007). These disputes led to the various waves of Arab immigration to the United States (Erickson & Al-Timimi, 2001).

The first wave of immigrants in the 1880s consisted of peasants and laborers who arrived in the United States in search of better economic opportunities (Haboush, 2007). Following this wave, for over 20 years between 1924 and 1947, the US government placed a restrictive quota on immigration for Arabs (Haboush, 2007). Then, after World War II, following the establishment of Israel in 1948, Palestinians who were displaced composed the majority of the second wave of immigration (Haboush, 2007). Finally, the third wave began in the 1960s and increased in 1975, as a result of Lebanese Civil War with the majority of immigrants consisting of highly educated professionals, as well as immigrants of the Muslim faith (Haboush, 2007).

Lebanese Christians, Egyptians, and Syrians encompass the largest percentages of Arab Americans (Ajrouch, 2000; de la Cruz & Brittingham, 2003), with most being second- and third-generation (Haboush, 2007). Although, more recent immigrants have arrived to the United States in response to the Iraq and Gulf wars (Haboush, 2007) and are likely to present with symptoms of posttraumatic stress disorder, have lower levels of education, fewer economic resources, and have more difficulty assimilating (Erickson & Al-Timimi, 2001; Nassar-McMillan & Hakim-Larson, 2003). Research indicates that Muslims may have more difficulty assimilating that Christians with the reason being that Christians tend to identify more strongly with Western culture and, perhaps, are less visible targets because of their Western dress (Nassar-McMillan & Hakim-Larson, 2003). Finally, levels of education and family income for Arab Americans are relatively higher than other immigrants (Brittingham & de la Cruz, 2005), which provides more opportunities for assimilation into American culture (Kulczycki & Lobo, 2002).

Religion

Haboush (2007) identified religion as one of the central factors of Arab cultures, as it permeates all aspects of the culture, including family life, child rearing, and educational and psychological views (Ajrouch, 2000). The significance of religion is to the point that identification with one's religious group often comes before identification with nationality (Haddad, 2002). Christianity and Islam are the two major religions that Arabs identify with (Nassar-McMillan & Hakim-Larson, 2003), although small numbers of other religious groups exist in Arab countries (e.g., Jews and Hindus; Haboush, 2007). According to Haboush (2007), the proportions of populations practicing each religion varies depending on the country: over 90% of the population in Syria, Egypt, Saudi Arabia, Qatar, Algeria, Bahrain, Jordan, Morocco, Libya, Tunisia, the United Arab Emirates, and Yemen are practicing Muslims, while Lebanon has historically been majority practicing Christians. Further, some Arab countries are governed by Islamic, or sharia, law, while other are sectarian (Haboush, 2007). Islam and Christianity are both integral to Arab culture. Therefore, religious values provide important sources for addressing and resolving problems (al-Krenawi & Graham, 2000; Hakim-Larson et al., 2007).

Arab Muslims. Contrary to common misconceptions, being Arab is not interchangeable with being Muslim, as Muslims are found in many countries throughout the world (Ali, Liu, & Humedian, 2004). The term "Islam" means "surrender" in Arabic, which in a religious context means "surrender to the will of Allah (God in Arabic)" (Haboush, 2007, p. 187). The term "Allah" is used by both Muslims and Christians in reference to God. The official religious text that Muslims follow is called the "Qu'ran," which was officially written in Arabic. Muslims believe that this text was handed down to the Prophet Mohammed from God in Saudi Arabia during the seventh century (Haboush, 2007). There are five pillars of Islam: the belief that there is only one God and that Mohammed is his Prophet; praying five times a day; giving charity to the needy; fasting during the holy month of Ramadan; and completing hajj, the pilgrimage to Mecca, if one has the health and financial means to do so (Ali et al., 2004). Islam divided into various sects throughout history—including Shiite, Sunni, Druze, and Alawi—with each sect having different religious beliefs, causing deep tensions among these subgroups (Haboush, 2007). Marriage between different subgroups is often discouraged in Arab culture (Erickson & Al-Timimi, 2001).

Arab Christians. Haboush (2007) identified the composition of Arab Christians, including Catholic, which encompasses Maronite, Greek, and Syrian Catholic; and non-Catholic groups who are primarily Orthodox consisting of Greek, Armenian, and Syrian Orthodox and Protestants. Historical divisions between Christians and Muslims are evident from the Maronites, who are Lebanese Christians, being the only Arab Christians to support the Crusades in fear of being taken over by Muslims (Haboush, 2005). The conflict between Maronites and Muslims eventually led to the Lebanese Civil War in 1975 (Haboush, 2007). Because of the historical tensions, intermarriage between Muslims and Christians is as much discouraged as is marriage between subgroups of the same religion (Haboush, 2007). As stated earlier, Arab Christians are more likely to identify with Western culture than Arab culture because of its association with Islam (Erickson & Al-Timimi, 2001). This is especially the case in Lebanon, as a result of the French rule and their protection of the Maronite Christians from 1920 until 1946 (Mackey, 1991).

Haboush (2007) highlighted the importance of understanding the religious conflicts and intergroup tensions discussed above when it comes to the school context in working with Arab American families. Due to these tensions, Arab individuals may present with attitudes of wariness and cautiousness toward other individuals who may be perceived as "outsiders." They may require some time to feel comfortable with school staff and trust them. Staff of European descent may have more difficulty establishing a working relationship with certain families due to the history of colonization and Western politics in the Middle East. This is further exacerbated by perceptions of the West being unsympathetic to and disinterested in Arab world views (Erickson & Al-Timimi, 2001). Even more complicating matters are the political events involving wars backed by the United States and economic sanctions imposed on Arab countries (Haboush, 2007).

Family

Haboush (2007) provided a general overview of family in Arab cultures. It is important to acknowledge that differences do exist among Arab countries but, in general, family is considered a central and unifying factor (Nassar-McMillan & Hakim-Larson, 2003). Regardless of religion, Arab culture is considered collectivist (Dwairy & Van Sickle, 1996), where the collective good of the family is critical in Arab society (Haboush, 2007). Growing up in a collectivist environment, Arabs tend to see themselves as members of groups rather than as individuals (Budman, Lipson, & Meleis, 1992). Budman et al. (1992) further indicate that cultural obligations require Arab adolescents shape themselves to conform to their family environments.

Family decisions are made with the objective of preserving family honor, stability, and cohesiveness (Haboush, 2007). For problem-solving, children are taught to utilize the family for solutions (al-Krenawi & Graham, 2000). Furthermore, children normally reside with their parents until marriage (al-Krenawi & Graham, 2000). Consequently, there is often stressful tensions in Arab American families between traditional collectivistic values and the individualistic values of contemporary American life (Hakim-Larson et al., 2007). Additionally, the extended family is a significant unit in Arab culture regardless of religion or nationality (Nydell, 2006). The common base for collectivistic family values stems from the followers of the ancient scriptures of the Abrahamic religions (Judaism, Christianity, and Islam) in the Middle East (Hakim-Larson et al., 2007).

Arab culture is also traditionally considered patriarchal (al-Krenawi & Graham, 2000; Erickson & Al-Timimi, 2001), where the father is the dominant authority and occasionally older brothers have some control over mothers and sisters (Haboush, 2007). Men are viewed as the main source of protection and provision for women (Hakim-Larson et al., 2007). Women are expected to uphold their conventional maternalistic roles of nurturing the emotional and domestic needs of men (Hakim-Larson et al., 2007). Generally, women's social roles are those of wife and mother, and unmarried women often remain living with their parents until marriage (Haboush, 2007). Even when the wife and mother contributes to family income and child discipline, she strives to preserve her husband's perception as head of the family (Budman et al., 1992). These roles are strengthened by traditions of Islam as well (Haboush, 2007). Worth noting is that very few Arab countries (i.e., Saudi Arabia) practice gender segregation in various public settings (Simmons, Simmons, & Habib Allah, 1994). Gender segregation is less commonly practiced among more acculturated families in the United States (Ajrouch, 2000). Therefore, when working with families, school staff need to convey respect for their values, even though they may be uncomfortable with patriarchal aspects of Arab culture (Dwairy & Van Sickle, 1996; Haboush, 2007). Further, where the family does uphold patriarchal traditions, developing an alliance with the father is critical to the success of establishing a trusting working relationship for any school purposes (al-Krenawi & Graham, 2000).

Haboush (2007) called on the development of visible alliances with the community and religious leaders to improve the understanding between school systems and Arab American communities. The author reported that families may express agreement with recommendations provided by schools for intervention with their child rather than voicing any opposition (al-Krenawi & Graham, 2000). The reason for this being that some Arab countries do not allow open opposition of their government. Some Arab families view schools as being an extension of the government and maintain this idea after immigrating (Haboush, 2007). Consequently, developing such alliances may serve as an intervention strategy systemically to strengthen relationships with Arab American families in schools (Nassar-McMillan & Hakim-Larson, 2003).

Perceptions of Education

Haboush (2007) indicated that education is highly valued for both boys and girls in Arab culture. Two primary reasons for this high regard include (Haboush, 2007): education's role in ensuring economic success for the family, enhancing the desirability of females for marriage, and the transmission of religious knowledge (Abu-saad, 1999; Ajrouch, 2000; Simmons et al., 1994). Additionally, for Muslims, the Qu'ran places a significant value on education; the holy book teaches them to continuously seek out knowledge and enlightenment throughout their lives (Al-Khatab,

1999). Therefore, Arab Americans tend to be more highly educated relative to the general American population (Brittingham & de la Cruz, 2005).

Haboush (2007) further noted that gender differences regarding education exist across Arab countries. The author compared the countries of Saudi Arabia and Lebanon as an example. In countries like Saudi Arabia, it was not until 1960 that females were allowed to access education. Furthermore, females are completely segregated from males (Simmons et al., 1994). It is important to note that education is valued for both males and females in these cases, but the reasoning behind it differs. While education for males is seen as a means for economic stability, for females it is seen as a means to increase desirability for marriage (Simmons et al., 1994). Comparatively, in Lebanon, educations for females has historically been more accessible and is more likely to lead to a profession (Haboush, 2007). In general, for men, education is perceived as ensuring economic stability for the family and are expected to contribute financially to extended family, according to Arab customs (Haboush, 2007; Mackey, 1991).

Various differences among Arab and American schools are also a factor, including instructional styles and strategies for behavior management (Haboush, 2007). Research shows that students in Arab schools have a less active role and, rather than development of critical thinking skills, Arab schools emphasize rote memorization of facts (e.g., Kibbi, 1995). Haboush (2007) added that, because Arab cultures tend to hold a high level of respect for authority figures and of their collectivist nature, parents hold high regard for teachers and allow them a great amount of control over their children. Further, upon immigration, Arab youth will have varying levels of English proficiency because the degree to which English is taught in schools varies across Arab countries (Haboush, 2007). Because of these various differences, Haboush (2007) suggested that more recent immigrants may benefit from a discussion regarding the differences between educational practices in the United States and Arab countries. The author posited that Arab American children may have difficulty adjusting to American school expectations to be active participants in questioning and debating ideas. Further, these students may appear to be passive because they do not understand the active role they are expected to demonstrate in their learning (Haboush, 2007). Discussions with parents and students regarding these differences and expectations may be critical to Arab American student success.

Haboush (2007) presented on the views of educational disabilities in Arab cultures. While many Arab countries have laws requiring education for youth with disabilities, families often keep their disabled children home in order to, culturally, avoid shame and dishonoring the family (Duvdevany & Abboud, 2003). For example, El Naggar Gaad (2001) conducted a study in the United Arab Emirates. The author found that mothers of children with Down's syndrome were more likely to place their children in residential or special schools rather than having them included in general education. Al Lawati (2011) indicated that persons with disabilities have been historically considered burdensome and shameful in Arab society. These attitudes certainly have a profound effect on families of persons with disabilities, not only preventing these individuals from receiving appropriate services but also making it difficult for them and their families to live a relatively normal life (Hadidi &

Al Khateeb, 2015). Al Lawati (2011) reported three major obstacles to special education services for youth with special needs in Arab countries:Firstly, some families are ashamed to acknowledge that their child is impaired or handicapped. Many children with mental disability are kept at home without receiving specialized services. Secondly, when families decide to seek placement for their children in either day centers or residential facilities, they may be faced with fees that they cannot afford given their poor financial conditions. Lastly, even after placing a child in a center, integrating the child later into society can be problematic. Not many schools accept children with a physical or mental handicap. Similarly, (and except for governmental agencies), few businesses will take on adolescents or young adults with special needs even though a specific job may be well within their capacity.

Hadidi and Al Khateeb (2015) provided an overview of the history of special education services in Arab countries. In a few countries, the first emergence occurred in the 1960s while others not until the 1980s or 1990s. There were four disability categories that were established by private and volunteer sectors: intellectual disabilities, hearing impairment, visual impairment, and physical disabilities. It was not until years later that government agencies became involved in special education services. In general, special education programs and services were based on charity and volunteer work (Hadidi, 1998). No formal training for teachers providing special education services was available until around the late 1970s. Higher education institutions began providing a 1-year or 2-year diploma in special education. Subsequently, some universities developed special education programs at the undergraduate and/or graduate levels. It was not until the 1990s that the majority of Arab countries began implementing laws for the "care and rehabilitation" of persons with disabilities and developed special education centers and schools (Hadidi & Al Khateeb, 2015, p. 520). Then, in 1994, with the release of the Salamanca Statement and Framework for Action on Special Needs Education by the United Nations Educational, Scientific, and Cultural Organization (UNESCO; UNESCO, 1994), Arab countries began reforming educational policies to promote inclusion of students with special educational needs into mainstream schools (Hadidi & Al Khateeb, 2015). Further, in 2006, the United Nations (UN) Convention on the Rights of Persons with Disabilities (UN, 2016) encouraged ensuring inclusive education systems at all levels of education (Hadidi & Al Khateeb, 2015). The proceedings from this convention led to the majority of Arab countries endorsing the idea of inclusive education and further moving to reform their educational systems to align with these measures (Hadidi & Al Khateeb, 2015).

While the idea of inclusive education is reportedly endorsed, putting it into practice is still essentially non-existent throughout the majority of Arab countries. There is no common strategy currently for special education services in Arab countries (Hadidi & Al Khateeb, 2015). The spectrum of services by each country ranges from segregation to inclusion at varying levels (Weber, 2012), with the majority following the segregation model (Hadidi & Al Khateeb, 2015). The field of special education has seen improvements over the past 30 years with government and non-government agencies and organizations working to protect the rights of persons with disabilities, improve educational opportunities for them, promote their independence and integration into society, and develop public awareness and education programs to improve their living conditions (Hadidi & Al Khateeb, 2015). Consequently, perceptions of disability and special education in Arab societies have become more positive (Hadidi & Al Khateeb, 2015). Persons with disabilities have become more visible members of their communities, and in turn, their struggles have become more normalized in public spheres (Hadidi & Al Khateeb, 2015). That being said, there continues to be a need for significant improvement in the special education sector in Arab countries.

Haboush (2007) warned school psychologists in particular to be aware that eligibility for special education may be associated with ethnic segregation for some families. For example, similar to the overrepresentation of minority youth relative to their proportion in the US population, Arab students in Israel are twice as likely to be diagnosed with intellectual disabilities as Jewish students (Dinero, 2002). Dinero (2002) reported that Israeli Arab students comprise 15–20% of elementary and secondary school populations but comprise 25–30% of the special education population. Further, they receive fewer educational services, have limited access to special education facilities, and are less likely to be mainstreamed than Israeli Jewish students (Dinero, 2002; Haboush, 2007). Consequently, for some Arab American families, such social-political contexts of special education practices in some Arab countries may cause an increased resistance to disability classification for special education (Haboush, 2007). Therefore, Haboush (2007) recommended framing educational objectives in a manner consistent with religious and cultural values.

Perceptions of Mental Health

Next, Haboush (2007) addressed views of mental health in Arab cultures. Factors such as attitudes toward mental health services and degree of familiarity with psychologists influence Arab American family's trust and acceptance of psychological services in the schools (Haboush, 2007). Research shows that psychology is closely associated with education in several Arab countries (Dwairy & Van Sickle, 1996), which may serve as a catalyst to the acceptance of mental health interventions in the schools (Haboush, 2007). In other Arab countries, however, serious mental illness is still associated with psychology (Hamdi, Amin, & Abou-Saleh, 1997; Soueif & Ahmed, 2001). Further, Arabs may be reluctant to admit having emotional problems in fear of dishonoring their family (al-Krenawi & Graham, 2000); mental illness is viewed as a social stigma that casts negative light on the family of the diagnosed individual (Budman et al., 1992; Gaines & Farmer, 1986). There is evidence that psychological issues are often expressed as somatic complaints (al-Krenawi & Graham, 2000; Budman et al., 1992), and therefore, Arabs are more likely to seek medical attention than psychological attention (Haboush, 2007; Nassar-McMillan & Hakim-Larson, 2003).

Research shows that posttraumatic stress disorder (PTSD) has been commonly found among immigrants exposed to regional wars or conflicts, for example, recent immigrants from Iraq (Haboush, 2007; Nassar-McMillan & Hakim-Larson, 2003). Therefore, school mental health providers need to assess whether a family's immigration was a result of war (Haboush, 2007). If this is the case, they need to assess whether the adolescent's school-related difficulties are related to possible PTSD (Haboush, 2007; Tatar & Horenczyk, 2003). Symptoms related to PTSD may potentially significantly impair adolescents' ability to concentrate in school (Al-Saffar, Borgå, Edman, & Hällström, 2003).

Mental health issues faced by Arab American youth are particularly associated with acculturation and discrimination (Goforth et al., 2017). Goforth et al. (2017) indicated that youth undergoing the acculturation process may have a stronger orientation toward their Arab heritage culture, toward the mainstream United States culture, or both cultures (bicultural). Goforth, Oka, Leong, and Denis (2014) demonstrated that the maintenance of Arab heritage cultural traditions was associated with fewer psychological problems in Muslim Arab American adolescents. Further, Goforth, Pham, Chun, Castro-Olivo, and Yosai (2016) found that higher levels of acculturative stress—defined as stress related to cultural adaptation—were associated with higher levels of internalizing symptoms, particularly among Muslims Arab American female adolescents. Acculturative stress is especially concerning during adolescence, as this is the time they are developing their identities and figuring out their societal roles (Goforth et al., 2017).

Another factor possibly influencing mental health in Arab American adolescents involves parent's acculturation status and parent–child relationship (Goforth et al., 2017). Goforth, Pham, and Oka (2015) found that acculturation gaps between Arab American parents and children predicted more behavioral problems in these adolescents. Further, the authors found that the association between adolescent acculturative stress and behavior problems was mediated by parent–child conflict. Therefore, it is important for school psychologists and counselors who provide mental health services in the schools to examine the extent of differences between parent and child acculturation levels and how that may be affecting the adolescent's mental health.

Cultural resources, such as strong ethnic identity, religious coping, and religious support, have been found to provide protection toward negative outcomes for Arab American adolescents (Ahmed, Kia-Keating, & Tsai, 2011; Goforth et al., 2017). For example, Goforth et al. (2016) showed that participation in organized religious practices was important for Muslim Arab American adolescents, while Ebstyne King and Furrow (2004) further indicated that the influence that religious participation has on adolescent behavior was mediated by trusting interactions with adults. Ethnic enclaves have also been identified as protective for Arab American adolescents (Kumar et al., 2014). Living in a community with others of similar ethnic or religious backgrounds may provide Arab American adolescents with more positive social support (Goforth et al., 2017).

Hakim-Larson et al. (2007) provided a comprehensive overview of considerations for mental health services with Arab Americans. Mental health interventions may be met with resistance because of the stigma of mental illness prevalent in more traditional families and/or those who have more recently immigrated (Abudabbeh, 2006). Factors that influence seeking treatment include shame, honor, dependence, family roles, and extent of acculturation (Hakim-Larson et al., 2007). In Arab culture, even throughout the various religions, the concept of "fate" exists and is a determining factor in seeking treatment, as individuals feel that there is little that can do to change the life situations they are in because it is predetermined by fate (Hakim-Larson et al., 2007; Nobles & Sciarra, 2000).

In providing mental health services for children in schools, it is important for school psychologists, counselors, and other mental health providers to first develop an alliance with the parents and demonstrate an empathic understanding that the parents have good intentions for their children before trying to implement any strategies to change parenting styles (Haboush, 2005; Hakim-Larson et al., 2007). This empathic relationship with parents should center their goals of putting family first and maintaining traditions and family honor (Hakim-Larson et al., 2007). Then, once they have a strong alliance, practitioners can attempt to demonstrate how some changes to mainstream culture can be made without sacrificing their goals (Hakim-Larson et al., 2007).

To further strengthen the relationship, mental health providers may consider conducting home visits in order to personalize their relationships and as a means of building rapport (Nassar-McMillan & Hakim-Larson, 2003). In developing rapport, hospitality and acceptance of food or beverage have been found useful (Haboush, 2005). Haboush (2007) emphasized the "deep-seated cultural tradition of hospitality," which allows this approach of socialization with the family to be more helpful in the initial rapport building journey than approaching with formalities right away (p. 192). All of the aforementioned strategies help focus on building the relationship first with Arab American families, which is absolutely critical before focusing on the problem and implementing any interventions (al-Krenawi & Graham, 2000; Hakim-Larson et al., 2007).

Haboush (2007) indicated that provision of mental health interventions is complicated by the fact that verbal expression of emotions/mental health is discouraged. The author suggested that school psychologists and other mental health providers pay close attention to the family's description of somatic complaints and religious explanations, as well as determine the extent to which the need to maintain family honor influences accurate reporting of potential psychological problems. Haboush (2007) further suggested the use of extended family members, when possible, to attend school meetings and help reinforce certain points presented.

As another consideration, Hakim-Larson et al. (2007) also noted the importance of gender for both client and clinician, especially with more traditional Muslim clients. Greetings of "hello" and "goodbye" are considered appropriate; however, handshakes with a woman may be considered inappropriate by a religious Muslim male (Hakim-Larson et al., 2007; Nydell, 2006). Furthermore, handshakes between a male and Muslim female are ultimately the woman's choice upon greeting or leaving (Nydell, 2006).

Process of Cultural Competence

Goforth et al. (2017) outlined the process of developing cultural competence for school-based mental health providers. This process may be utilized by all school staff working with Arab American youth. There are three main steps toward culturally competence practices: self-awareness, cultural knowledge, and skills to provide culturally responsive practice (Goforth et al., 2017). Questions that school professionals should ask themselves throughout each of these stages are presented in Table 2 (Goforth et al., 2017) and may be referred to for each of the next sections.

Table 2 Questions to consider in developing culturally responsive school-based mental health services for Arab American youths (Goforth et al., 2017)

Awareness	Knowledge	Skills
What is my own cultural background?	Is my school a positive, supportive place for all students, including Arab American students? If not, what aspects of the school could be improved?	What evidence-based treatments are available that would align with my client's goals?
What are my values and norms that shape my thoughts and behavior?	If my client is Muslim, what aspects of Islam should I learn about that is relevant for assessment or treatment?	What are their cultural considerations when choosing a particular treatment?
What are my biases about Arab Americans and/or Muslim Americans? What stereotypes do I currently hold and from where did I learn them?	What specific information do I need to gather about my Arab American client?	In what ways can I use non-discriminatory assessment with Arab American youths who are English-language learners?
How comfortable am I in providing mental health services to this Arab American client? What are the reasons why I might feel discomfort?	Are there any cultural brokers that could help me learn more about my client?	Are there particular professional training opportunities to help me provide services to Arab American youths?
What aspects of privilege do I hold? How does this privilege affect my practice in school-based mental health services?	Is there information I need to gather about Arab history (e.g., Arab–Israeli conflict) that would allow me to support my client better?	Do the norms of the mental health measures that I use include Arab Americans? If there are none that meet the requirements, to what degree do I trust the assessment results?

Step 1: Self-Awareness

In schools, it is up to staff to serve as catalysts for change in the student environment. Before change can begin, school staff need to examine their own beliefs and stereotypes for they cannot promote systemic change when they hold stereotypes against different cultures (Devine, Forscher, Austin, & Cox, 2012). Awareness begins with critical self-reflection and an understanding that cultural competence is a life-long process (Goforth et al., 2017). Through critical self-reflection, school professionals may become aware of their own biases and stereotypes they hold related to Arab American cultures (Goforth et al., 2017), which then leads to increased openness about working with Arab American youth in schools (Goforth, 2016).

Step 2: Cultural Knowledge

School professionals should develop knowledge regarding Arab American cultures, values, religious beliefs, and language (Goforth et al., 2017). Goforth et al. (2017) presented various books and resources about Arab American cultures that can be utilized in learning about these factors, which can be found in Table 1. The authors also suggested collaborating with cultural consultants to provide information about cultural norms and values when working with various Arab American youth and their families. As stated earlier in this chapter, the heterogeneity of this population makes it impossible to generalize these characteristics (Goforth et al., 2017), so it is critical to be aware of any differences that exist in the norms and values of individual families.

Many school staff continue to report a lack of knowledge regarding Arab cultures (Haboush & Alyan, 2016). For example, Aburumuh, Smith, and Ratcliffe (2009) examined the environment of an entire school district in San Antonio, Texas to determine how much staff actually knew about the Arab and Islamic cultures. The theoretical framework used was Care Theory, which posits that "caring educators move beyond superficial or technical concerns and attempt to engage students in meaningful activities that validate their culture, language, and perspectives while supporting their academic and emotional needs" (Aburumuh et al., 2009, p. 11). The authors used a questionnaire called the Educators' Cultural Awareness and Perceptions (E-CAP), which presented two sets of questions that focused on the basic terminology for these two cultures that are commonly misused and misapplied. The authors found that the educators in this district had limited understanding of both Arab and Muslim children, which lead to erroneous assumptions, pernicious beliefs, negative stereotypes, and, ultimately, barriers to students' education. Therefore, when it comes to the students, no matter race and ethnicity, staff need to be sure that they understand the cultures they are working with so they are providing effective services. Once school staff start learning about other cultures, they can start developing deeper and more meaningful relationships with their students. As Abu El-Haj (2006) states, "educators are encouraged to learn about the cultural traditions, values, customs, and norms of the communities from which their students come to be able to interact with students and families in culturally appropriate ways" (pp. 23). Perhaps schools can start with a similar activity to obtain an overall measure of misperceptions and use this information to determine what cultural training program to implement to gain knowledge of Arab American cultures.

Step 3: Culturally Relevant Skill Set

School professionals should develop a skill set to provide culturally responsive practices to Arab American populations (Goforth et al., 2017). For teachers, this can be the use of culturally relevant teaching, which will be discussed later in this chapter. For school psychologists and other school-based mental health providers, this is related to culturally responsive assessments and evidence-based treatments (Goforth et al., 2017). Mental health providers may utilize professional development and cultural consultation in developing skills in non-discriminatory assessment, working with English language learners, and, as mentioned earlier in this chapter, home–school collaboration with Arab American families to increase rapport building (Goforth et al., 2017). School professionals may also utilize training opportunities through universities or professional organizations to develop culturally appropriate skills (Goforth et al., 2017).

Intercultural Relations with Peers and Staff

Protecting students from experiencing discrimination in schools involves promoting activities that foster more positive interracial climates and better intergroup relations (Benner & Graham, 2013). Examples include cooperative learning programs that allow youth to establish a common in-group identity (Gaertner & Dovidio, 2000) and extracurricular activities that encourage interracial mixing (Clotfelter, 2002). Perhaps the single most important strategy to strengthen social support for Arab American students in schools is increasing the awareness of the culture itself in the school systems and countering negative stereotypes (Tabbah, Miranda, & Wheaton, 2016). School staff need to assess acts of intolerance to determine if they are related to a lack of cultural understanding from peers. School professionals may take numerous actions to counter a lack of cultural understanding. For instance, school practitioners can facilitate the development of multi-ethnic group organizations that focus on peer members teaching about their cultures/ethnic groups and learning about others (Tabbah, Miranda, & Wheaton, 2016; Wingfield, 2006). Najjar et al. (2019) stated that formal activities of cultural expression within the school setting may reduce barriers for Arab American and other cultural youth to educate others about their heritage. Focus groups may be held during lunchtime, free periods, or after school. As members of these organizations, students may be encouraged to immerse themselves in multicultural activities to explore other ethnicities and cultures. Such focus groups in schools can serve as a catalyst in building strong social support; students can learn from each other and begin to respect each other's differences. Staff may, in turn, learn about the source of conflict between students and whether it has to do anything with cultural misunderstandings.Barrett (2018) provided specific strategies for schools to promote the intercultural competence of students, based on a review of existing literature. The author first explained what intercultural competence entails and then outlined the various actions that schools can take to encourage development of intercultural competence. Barrett (2018) defined intercultural competence as:

> The set of values, attitudes, skills, knowledge, and understanding that are needed for understanding and respecting people who are perceived to be culturally different from oneself, for interacting and communicating effectively and appropriately with such people, and for establishing positive and constructive relationships with such people. (p. 94)[1]

Barrett (2018) posited that various human interactions occur in everyday life at an interpersonal level without much thought of cultural differences. There are situations, however, when cultural differences become salient, which then causes an individual to shift their frame of reference from interpersonal to intercultural (Barrett, 2018). The author identified five conditions that can lead to this type of shift:

- When there are perceptually salient cultural signs, emblems, or practices present that serve to elicit the cultural category in the mind of the individual.
- When cultural categories are frequently used by the individual to think about other people, so that these categories are primed and are readily accessed by that individual when he or she interacts with, or perceives, other people.
- When cultural categories help the individual to make sense of the pattern of similarities and differences between the people who are present within a situation.
- When cultural categories help the individual to make sense of why another person is behaving in the way that they are.
- When the individual's own cultural affiliations are experienced as being disadvantaged, devalued, discriminated against, or threatened in some other way by the cultural group to which the other person is perceived as belonging. (p. 94)[2]

When a situation shifts from interpersonal to intercultural in this manner, an individual does not respond to the other individual on the basis of their own individual characteristics, rather on the basis of their cultural affiliations (Barrett, 2018). Therefore, Barrett (2018) indicated that, when a shift like this occurs due to

[1] Used with permission from *European Psychologist* (2018), 23(1), 93–104. ©2018 Hogrefe Publishing www.hogrefe.comhttps://doi.org/10.1027/1016-9040/a000308

[2] Used with permission from *European Psychologist* (2018), 23(1), 93–104. ©2018 Hogrefe Publishing www.hogrefe.comhttps://doi.org/10.1027/1016-9040/a000308

perceived cultural differences that have occurred from any of the above situations or by the individual's own psychological or cultural orientation, intercultural competence becomes especially relevant. The author suggested that these intercultural situations apply to children from the time they start attending school. The reason being that research has shown that children begin classifying others into ethnic and racial categories as early as 3–4 years of age, and they make intergroup comparisons and attitudes almost immediately after (Barrett & Buchanan-Barrow, 2011). Further, between the ages of 3 and 5 years, children begin to classify others into national groups and make similar comparisons and develop attitudes toward them (Barrett, 2007).

Researchers agree that the main components of intercultural competence include values, attitudes, skills, and knowledge and critical understanding (Barrett, 2016, 2018; Deardorff, 2006). Barrett (2016) further identified what each of these components encompass: *Values* consist of valuing human dignity and human rights, and valuing cultural diversity; *Attitudes* involve openness to cultural otherness and to other beliefs, worldviews, and practices, respect for other people and for other beliefs, worldviews, and practices, self-efficacy, and tolerance of ambiguity; *Skills* are composed of analytical and critical thinking skills, skills of listening and observing, empathy, flexibility and adaptability, and linguistic, communicative, and plurilingual skills; and, *knowledge and critical understanding* involves knowledge and critical understanding of the self, knowledge and critical understanding of language and communication, and knowledge and critical understanding of culture, cultures, and religions. (Barrett, 2018, p. 95)[3]

Barrett (2018) suggested that several of these components can be addressed as early as preschool and primary school, whereas others are at a higher developmental level. The author called on the schools to implement activities in the school system to help promote and foster these skills in students. Barrett (2018) outlined three major actions that schools can take including intergroup contact, pedagogical approaches, and school institutional policies.

Schools can promote intercultural competence through actions based on intergroup contact (Barrett, 2018). First, they can encourage intercultural friendships among students, which may reduce prejudice toward individuals from other cultural groups (Barrett, 2018; Pettigrew & Tropp, 2006). It is not enough for students from different cultural backgrounds just to have contact with each other. Rather, cooperation and collaborative efforts are required among students, in which they must have common goals and see themselves as having equal status with each other (Barrett, 2018). Intergroup contact and friendships should be explicitly encouraged in school policies, which teachers should explicitly endorse (Barrett, 2018). Barrett (2018) defined four conditions that should be met to maximize effects:

- The contact should take place between people who perceive themselves to be of equal status within the contact situation.

[3]Used with permission from *European Psychologist* (2018), 23(1), 93–104. ©2018 Hogrefe Publishing www.hogrefe.comhttps://doi.org/10.1027/1016-9040/a000308

- The contact should be sufficiently prolonged and close that it has the potential to allow meaningful relationships or friendships to develop between the participants.
- The contact should involve cooperation on joint activities that are aimed at achieving common goals (rather than competition between groups).
- The contact should be backed by an explicit framework of support by those in authority or by social institutions. (p. 96)[4]

Research demonstrates that intercultural competence can also be developed among youth using indirect intergroup contact (Barrett, 2018; Turner & Cameron, 2016), including imaginative contact (Stathi, Cameron, Hartley, & Bradford, 2014; Turner, West, & Christie, 2013) and extended contact (Cameron, Rutland, Douch, & Brown, 2006). Additionally, intergroup contact may be encouraged through the organization of study abroad programs for students (Barrett, 2018). Research shows that students who participate in such programs gain higher levels of intercultural competence, have lower levels of anxiety when interacting with individuals from other cultures, and hold more friendships with individuals from different cultures (Hammer, 2004). The downfall of this is that the school and students need to have the financial ability to be able to participate in such programs (Barrett, 2018). In such cases, an alternative could be arranging for students to have Internet-based cultural contact (Barrett, 2018; Barrett, Byram, Lázár, Mompoint-Gaillard, & Philippou, 2013; Fisher, Evans, & Esch, 2004). Examples provided by Barrett (2018) included online video conferencing and social media for collaborative projects between students in different countries or different regions of the same country, where students can introduce themselves, interview each other, discuss various issues, and complete tasks designated by teachers. These types of activities can, according to Barrett (2018), foster the development of "openness, listening skills, perspective-taking skills, tolerance of ambiguity, respect for others, critical thinking skills, and critical understanding of culture and cultures" (p. 98). For Arab American students, programs such as AMIDEAST provide various resources with their mission being "to create hope, opportunity, and mutual understanding among people in the Middle East, North Africa, and the United States through life-changing opportunities for education and cultural exchanges" (www.amideast.org). This resource may be useful in preparing study abroad programs and/or online intercultural interactions as discussed by Barrett (2018).

Another activity for intercultural contact involves the development of educational connections and partnerships with organizations and individuals in the community (Barrett, 2018). Individuals from various cultural backgrounds can be invited to the school to perform various classroom activities. Students can also attend field trips to community and religious organizations in their neighborhood (Barrett, 2018). Activities may involve interviews, observations, and critical reflections regarding cultural differences (Barrett, 2018). For Arab American students,

---

[4]Used with permission from *European Psychologist* (2018), 23(1), 93–104. ©2018 Hogrefe Publishing www.hogrefe.comhttps://doi.org/10.1027/1016-9040/a000308

teachers and administrators may invite Arab American speakers to the schools to speak, show films, and help with cultural exhibits (Wingfield, 2006). These community members may be accessed by school librarians to ask for recommendations for new school library resources (Wingfield, 2006). Additionally, various Arab American organizations offer services to schools for the development of cultural competence (Wingfield, 2006). Resources and organizations cited by Wingfield (2006, p. 263) that continue to be available to the public and may be used by educators in organizing intercultural activities for their students include: *Al-Jadid*, a magazine of Arab culture, literature, and the arts (http://www.aljadid.com/); *Mizna*, a journal of Arab American literature and promotes Arab culture (http://mizna.org); Teachers may also access Middle East study centers at universities that have developed their own resources and training workshops for K-12 teachers. For example, the Center for Contemporary Arab Studies at Georgetown University has a K-14 educational outreach program for teachers (https://ccas.georgetown.edu/resources/k-14-outreach/). For over 40 years, the program had provided—and continues to provide—professional development for teachers throughout the country to help develop their knowledge about the diverse cultures, histories, and religions of the Middle East and North Africa from a global perspective. They provide workshops and institutes, teaching units and background modules, assistance with curriculum development, and a lending library. The program also offers an Education Outreach email list for educators to join to receive notifications of upcoming events and information regarding new teaching materials and other opportunities for teachers; The Middle East Institute has online materials for educators to access (http://www.mideasti.org); In addressing Islam, teachers may utilize the Council on American/Islamic Relations (www.cair-net.org) and the Muslim Public Affairs Committee (http://www.mpac.org) for sources of information on Muslim civil rights issues; The Council on Islamic Education offers teacher guides to Islam and to teaching about Islam in the public school and other resources (http://www.cie.org). These guides are available to download free of charge; Dar al Islam is "a non-profit organization dedicated to cultivating greater understanding of Islam among Americans in order to establish our commonalities and build stronger relationships" (http://www.daralislam.org). This organization offers resources for educators to learn about Islam including a teacher's institute (http://www.daralislam.org/programs/education/teachers-institutes.aspx), which is also free of charge. Another organization that offers curriculum downloads free of charge, as well as training and other resources for educators on Islam, is Creating Cultural Competencies (Triple-C), which is a collaborative effort between the College of Education at the University of Illinois-Chicago and the American Friends Service Committee-Chicago (https://www.creatingculturalcompetencies.org/). The Triple-C initiative is to counter anti-Muslim racism and Islamophobia in schools. Additional resources are provided in Table 1 (Goforth et al., 2017).

The next category identified by Barrett (2018) was the promotion of intercultural competence through pedagogical approaches. These approaches include the encouragement of students' critical reflection on their intercultural experiences and their own cultural identities, cooperative learning activities, and project-based learning.

Barrett (2018) suggested two educational tools specifically developed by Barrett and colleagues to support their critical reflections on intercultural experiences and their own identities: the Autobiography of Intercultural Encounters (Byram, Barrett, Ipgrave, Jackson, & Méndez García, 2009) and the Autobiography of Intercultural Encounters through Visual Media (Barrett, Byram, Ipgrave, & Seurrat, 2013). All required documents and activities for these educational tools can be found online free for download (https://www.coe.int/en/web/autobiography-intercultural-encounters). Barrett, Byram, Lázár, et al. (2013) suggest additional strategies, including activities emphasizing multiple perspectives; role plays and simulations; analyzing texts, films, and plays; and ethnographic tasks, which involve students observing or talking to people outside of the classroom and then returning to the classroom with notes that they can compare and reflect upon critically.

Finally, Barrett (2018) identified activities to promote intercultural competence through school institutional policies. These actions include utilizing culturally inclusive and relevant curriculum and adopting a whole school approach to valuing diversity and human rights. Research shows that the inclusion of culturally inclusive curricula helps reduce students' cultural prejudices and fosters a greater sense of respect for different cultures (Ladson-Billings, 1992). At the whole school level, valuing diversity and human rights can be expressed at all levels through "teaching and learning methods, leadership, governance, school decision-making structures and policies, codes of behavior, interpersonal relationships including staff-student relationships, extracurricular activities, and external links to the community" (Barrett, 2018, p. 101). The next section focuses on how these two actions may be implemented in schools for Arab American adolescents.

Educational Policy: Addressing Arabs and Arab Americans in Multicultural Curricula

In today's ever-growing world of diversity, a multicultural education is crucial in preparing and encouraging students "to live, learn, communicate, and work to achieve common goals in a culturally diverse world" (Crockett & Brown, 2009, p. 118). Arslan (2009) posited that, while administrative support is important to the development of teachers' multicultural education endeavors, educational policy is key in implementation and maintenance of multiculturalism. A multicultural curriculum at all school levels including staff and students allows for all members to develop an understanding of their society and all cultures of the world (Arslan, 2009). The National Education Association (NEA;, 2008) identified three policy levers that can help educators develop cultural competence including preservice education, licensure, and ongoing professional development. The NEA (2008) emphasized the importance of preservice education training in cultural competence and noted that currently only one-third of the United States offers diversity training in their educational programs. Having such training in place and ensuring that the

Arab American culture is included and accurately represented are critical steps for policymakers.

Concerning Arab American cultures, Wingfield (2006) discussed the problem of it being inexistent or an inaccurate inclusion in curriculum development. The culture is often represented in a superficial manner or through political context (Wingfield, 2006). The literature shows striking evidence that this was the case with the samples being investigated regarding curriculum content on Arab cultures. For example, Tabbah (2016) investigated this in particular and found that the majority of the student sample reported that Arab American culture was either not represented at all or misrepresented in the multicultural paradigm in their schools. Additionally, Najjar et al. (2019) found that a lack of representation, misrepresentation, or exclusively negative representation of Arab history and culture was a source of acculturative stress on Arab American youth and that this may push students to either distance themselves from their heritage or engage in cognitive and emotional labor to rectify these presentations of the culture and history in the curriculum. This in and of itself is a problem and can affect feelings of belonging.

School systems need to thoroughly examine the cultures of students enrolled and make sure they are included in the multicultural paradigm. Not only do they need to be represented, but schools also need to be aware of the accuracy of the materials being taught regarding different cultures, races, ethnicities, and religions. One of the sources of discrimination found in the research is the lack of and/or misrepresentation of Arab cultures in the multicultural curriculum. Wingfield (2006) delved further and suggests that the decision that teachers make on what to include and what to avoid is a source of discrimination:Arab and Muslim issues may be seen as "complex," too "controversial," or too "dangerous." The Palestinian issue is one of special sensitivity. Its presence or absence and the way it is addressed in the classroom are often shaped by the dominance of pro-Israeli perspectives in the United States and among educators. Judgments as to what is "controversial" may be a measure of the relative political power of the Arab-American and Jewish communities to influence what is considered legitimate and "mainstream" discourse within school systems. Palestinian viewpoints are often excluded or marginalized. Until a Palestinian viewpoint is introduced, Israeli-centric views are not considered "controversial." The essential question though is not the ethnicity or religion of decision-makers. Jewish educators are often among those most attuned and responsive to Palestinian perspectives. The issue is the ideologies and mindsets that shape the decisions that are made. Basic justice demands that Arab voices and perspectives be heard on issues that involve them. (p. 258)

To counter this problem, Wingfield (2006) provided an invaluable guide to help schools in the transformation of curriculum and instruction to integrate Arab American ethnic content. The guide incorporated Banks' (2003) four phases of multicultural infusion of ethnic content in the curriculum and applies it to Arab American ethnic content. The four phases include contributions, ethnic additions, transformation, and social action (Banks, 2003). Wingfield (2006) presented how Arab American ethnic content can be incorporated at each phase.

At the contributions phase, schools would include heroes, holidays, and artifacts of Arab American cultures (Wingfield, 2006). Resources provided throughout this chapter, including Table 1 (Goforth et al., 2017) may be utilized in researching the various ethnic content relevant to this phase. Some examples provided by Wingfield (2006), however, may include figures such as Helen Thomas, former dean of the White House press corps, and other famous Arab Americans such as Casey Kasem and Tony Shalhoub. The author suggested possibly holding a matching exercise on "Famous Arab Americans" that could defy stereotypes (p. 260). In terms of holidays, Wingfield (2006) noted that the lack of recognition of Muslim holidays for Muslim Arab students in schools, given that other religious holidays such as Christmas and Hanukkah are recognized, leads to them feeling the inequity. Therefore, inclusion of Muslim holidays on the official school calendar is critical in the contributions phase. Further, schools should consider holding events to honor Arab American students and families, as well as special classes, exhibits, and, when possible, field trips to churches, mosques, or community organizations to learn more about Arab cultures (Wingfield, 2006).

The next phase is ethnic additions to the curriculum (Wingfield, 2006). Wingfield (2006) stated that Arab American ethnic content can be added to the curriculum without changing its basic structure, including courses on American history, literature, music, food, civics, and social studies. These are all areas that Arab Americans have contributed to throughout their immigration history in the United States. This phase is considered more of a superficial phase according to Wingfield (2006). The author states that attention to Arab American concerns can only be truly addressed in a restructured curriculum, hence, the transformative phase of curriculum change. What is truly needed is the "systematic and conscious inclusion of Arab Americans in every aspect of the curriculum and in school life more broadly" (p. 261). This, then, becomes a matter for school institutional policy to address comprehensively (Wingfield, 2006). Wingfield (2006) identified a significant barrier in this transformative phase as being the level at which educators have internalized multicultural values. In the case of Arab American ethnic content, for true transformative change, educators must have a certain degree of political courage and tolerance for controversy (Wingfield, 2006). It requires educators to take a different perspective: the perspective of their Iraqi American students being concerned about their families in Baghdad during the Gulf wars (Wingfield, 2006), or the perspective Palestinian American families who discuss their history of being displaced from Palestine after the creation of Israel in 1948 (Wingfield, 2006), without thinking the former as being a "terrorist" or the latter as being "anti-Semitic." Therefore, in order for true transformation, educators need to be seriously willing to address political issues (Wingfield, 2006), which comes along with the development of true cultural competence, as stated early a genuine internalization of multicultural values (Wingfield, 2006), and desire for social justice. Resources listed previously by Wingfield (2006) and Table 1 (Goforth et al., 2017) may be utilized for this phase and in the development of multicultural competence for educators. Brief examples for transformative action provided by Wingfield (2006) include the teachings of the diversity within the Arab world and Islam; teaching basics of Islam and discussing the frequent stereotypes about Muslims (e.g., Islam and violence, women in Islam, jihad, the position of Christians and Jews, Islam and democracy); making clear that the terrorists of 9/11 do not represent the Arab/Arab American mainstream or Muslim/Muslim American mainstream; building collaborative networks between school and Arab American communities, where schools can arrange for speakers to come and discuss various issues and address existing stereotypes. Ultimately, transformative action needs to move beyond addressing the existing stereotypes. The ultimate goal in this case is having representation of Arab culture that illuminates the beauty of the culture, as well as representation of Arab people just living their lives, outside of the context of war or ethnicity or anything stereotypically associated with them.

The fourth and final phase is social action and social justice, which calls for solidarity with Arab American and Muslim communities (Wingfield, 2006). Wingfield (2006) indicated that this can be accomplished by speaking out when racist attitudes are expressed, reaffirming school anti-discrimination policies, and publicly sending messages of support. Schools should contact friends in the community or Arab American organizations and mosques to request support during times of crises (Wingfield, 2006). Discrimination incidents in the schools should be used as learning experiences for staff and students and opportunities to strengthen relations between groups (Wingfield, 2006). Panels of individuals from the Arab American community can be invited to address school staff and/or students, depending on the type of incident, regarding cultural perceptions (Wingfield, 2006). In addition, schools can facilitate student groups that address issues of anti-discrimination and diversity (Wingfield, 2006).

Haboush and Alyan (2016) stated that the current national education standards include sections on discrimination and teaching tolerance. Therefore, they suggested that these segments should be incorporated in classroom instruction regarding 9/11. Sabry and Bruna (2007) called for schools to have an ongoing dialogue with parents to verify the accuracy and appropriateness of instructional material being presented on Arab American cultures in the classroom. A combination of these resources may help counter discrimination in schools by informing educators and students about Arab American cultures.

Moreover, teacher expectations for students may be influenced by their misinformation about Arab cultures (Haboush & Alyan, 2016). Teachers may perpetuate this misinformation unintentionally through biased and inaccurate teaching practices (Haboush & Alyan, 2016; Sabry & Bruna, 2007). In turn, students may set low expectations for themselves regarding their academic performance if they have no suitable cultural role models to identify with along with low teacher expectations (Haboush & Alyan, 2016). School practitioners and administrators may work with teachers to address inaccurate expectations and help search for resources to provide them with skill-building in cultural competence pertaining to Arab American students (Haboush & Alyan, 2016). Resources in Table 1 may facilitate this, as well as the resources listed above from Wingfield (2006).Along similar lines, practitioners may facilitate training in culturally-responsive teaching (Gay, 2000). Founded by Ladson-Billings (1992):Culturally relevant teaching serves to empower students to the point where they will be able to examine critically educational content and process and ask what its role is in creating a truly democratic and multicultural society. It uses the students' culture to help them create meaning and understand the world. Thus, not only academic success, but social and cultural success are emphasized by the culturally relevant teacher. (p. 106)

According to Gay (2000), culturally responsive teaching, among various other attributes, acknowledges the legitimacy of the cultural heritages of different ethnic groups, and it teaches students to understand and praise their own and others' cultural backgrounds. In the process of such training, it is critical to have representative and accurate information regarding various cultures. Swindler Boutte and Hill (2006) suggested seeking advice from African American communities to inform best practices for teaching students of color. Similar methods may be applied with Arab American communities. Practitioners may facilitate teachers' exploration of the different systems involved in the lives of their Arab American students and use the information to develop culturally relevant pedagogies. Ultimately, this type of teaching enables the elimination of misconceptions regarding Arab American cultures in the classrooms and, subsequently, perhaps, mainstream society. This allows students to thrive, as well, and validates their experiences and allows the entire class community to thrive.

Intervention for Developmental Outcomes in Schools: Multiple-Tiered Systems of Support

Attaining a strong ethnic identity is important developmentally. However, exposure to various forms of discrimination may prevent adolescents from developing a healthy sense of acculturation and may cause them to have difficulty integrating with society (Hakim-Larson & Menna, 2016). When young individuals are treated differently by the dominant culture, they potentially respond by defending their cultural integrity. However, researchers have found discrimination to be the most important barrier to assimilation for immigrants (Stepick & Stepick, 2002). Wray-Lake, Syvertsen, and Flanagan (2008), in their study including Arab American adolescents, suggested that these negative experiences might make it difficult for Arab American youth to identify with being an American citizen. The authors suggested that these adolescents have to learn what it means to be American through "the context of negative images of their ethnic group" (Wray-Lake et al., 2008, p. 91). Therefore, when providing school-based mental health services, practitioners working with Arab American adolescents must evaluate and incorporate their experiences and developmental outcomes in counseling assessment and intervention; clinicians must consider the adolescent's cultural context as well as the development of the adolescent within their cultural context (Jones, 2009). Goforth et al. (2017) provided a general framework for school-based mental health providers to reference when providing services using multi-tiered systems of support. Multi-tiered systems of support (MTSS) is designed to address the individual needs of

Table 3 Recommendations for multi-tiered systems of support for Arab American youths (Goforth et al., 2017)

Tier level	Recommended services
Tier I: Universal services	• Screen all students for mental health issues • Develop and implement prevention programs to reduce likelihood of mental health issues • Provide culturally inclusive curricula that fairly and accurately represent Arabs, the Middle East, and Muslims (Schwartz, 2002) • Provide professional development opportunities for teachers to learn about Arab American students (Carter & El Hindi, 1999)
Tier II: Targeted intervention and services	• Consider how family should be involved in all aspects of school-based services when a student is found at-risk for internalizing or externalizing symptoms • Take into account how Arab American youths may present their symptoms through physical symptoms or somatic terms (Melhem & Chemali, 2014) • Recognize how acculturative stress may be affecting students struggling with their heritage (i.e., Arab) and/or mainstream (i.e., American) cultures • Examine the advantages and disadvantages of group counseling while considering the family and culture
Tier III: Intensive intervention and special education services	• Provide comprehensive, non-discriminatory assessment of the students' mental health and academic performance. The assessment should include a clinical interview, observation, language proficiency, and standardized norm-based measures (Rhodes, Ochoa, & Ortiz, 2005) • Establish alliances with the family and integrate the family into interventions or counseling • Ensure that individualized interventions are chosen that are culturally appropriate and take into account factors, such as collective trauma and family/community relationships

each student and, in terms of school-based mental health services, involves three tiers which increase in levels of intensity at each tier: Tier I involves mental health services provided at a universal level for all students; Tier II involves a targeted group of students with moderate needs; and Tier III involves individuals with very specific needs requiring intensive intervention (Goforth et al., 2017). The next section discusses the recommendations cited by Goforth et al. (2017) at each tier, although the authors caution practitioners from assuming the uniformity of Arab American experiences. A summary of recommendations is also provided in Table 3 (Goforth et al., 2017).

Tier I of MTSS involves screening all students for mental health problems and providing them with comprehensive, school-wide programs to prevent mental health issues from developing (Goforth et al., 2017). The research shows that school climate is one of the most important factors in mental health prevention, since a positive school climate allows students to feel a sense of safety (Cohen, McCabe,

Michelli, & Pickeral, 2009). Moreover, a school climate that is accepting of cultural diversity and intolerant of discrimination may provide Arab American adolescents with a healthier means of socialization without the stressors of discriminatory experiences. For example, Brown and Chu (2012) found that Mexican immigrant children with teachers who highly valued diversity held stronger ethnic identities and lower perceptions of discrimination than with teachers who devalued diversity. It is crucial to the development of adolescents for school professionals to examine the school environment and implement interventions where tolerance is lacking. Consequently, future research endeavors need to address school climate, as well as in practice and policy. According to Wingfield (2006) regarding K-12 atmosphere:A focus on culture helps replace the negative images of Arabs and Muslims generated by political and military conflicts, putting a human face on people too often thought discussed in terms of hostile stereotypes. It makes a difference when Arab American and Muslim children see their community and culture, and their parents, validated by the authority figures in their school (p. 260).

Examining school climate can begin by the process of cultural self-assessment at the individual, classroom-wide, school-wide, and system-wide levels (Crockett & Brown, 2009). The first step to developing cultural competence is developing a cultural self-awareness. Continuous objective feedback regarding cultural self-assessment is crucial in successful development of cultural awareness with the use of various procedures and tools (Crockett & Brown, 2009). Jones (2009) suggested several tools for individual cultural self-awareness for the purposes of counseling skills and intervention in the school system. First, increased self-awareness can begin through the use of the *Self-Assessment Checklist for Personnel Providing Services and Supports to Children and Their Families* (Goode, 2002). Practitioners may additionally develop a cultural genogram—a family tree that represents culture and diversity—to determine how culture and diversity has influenced their family history. Cultural self-awareness can also be cultivated through the use of journaling as a tool to reflect on their own biases and personal reactions toward clients that may affect the professional relationship. Finally, the author suggests the formation of diverse consulting groups with colleagues with whom to engage in regular dialogue about multicultural issues in counseling.

Kumar, Karabenick, Warnke, Hany, and Seay (2019) found that, within school policy, cultural responsiveness included teacher attitudes and beliefs regarding culturally diverse students and intergroup relationships with peers. Students in their study, which included a large number of Arab American adolescents, viewed their teachers attitudes and beliefs being empathetic, respectful, and interested and open to other cultures as more important and authentic than their actual cultural fluency (Kumar et al., 2019). Consequently, to assess the cultural responsiveness and inclusive learning environments, schools may utilize the Culturally Inclusive and Responsive Curricular Learning Environments (CIRCLEs; Kumar et al., 2019). The CIRCLEs features include cultural inclusiveness across academic disciplines for all students; teachers and school personnel who demonstrate cultural sensitivity, awareness, and cultural openness; culturally responsive school policies and practices; and the promotion and maintenance of positive intergroup relations among students who feel they matter, that their voice is heard, and that they belong (Kumar et al., 2019). The CIRCLEs measure encompasses the school environment as a whole and provides for all students curricular relevance across disciplines (Kumar et al., 2019). It also identifies and prioritizes teachers, administrators, and other school personnel who are culturally sensitive; encourages culturally responsive school practices and policy; and emphasizes the instances in which a school culture promotes positive intergroup relations and sense of belonging (Kumar et al., 2019). Since Arab/Arab American adolescents were included in their sample, the CIRCLEs may be deemed appropriate for use in measuring their perspectives of the school environment.

Once they start learning about other cultures, school professionals can begin appreciating, respecting, and cultivating more meaningful relationships with their students. Practitioners may be leaders in such activities in the school system. They would need to understand the cultures of the students/clients they are working with to ensure the provision of effective services in schools (Artiles & Ortiz, 2012). The next step is increasing "other" awareness, also known as increasing cultural literacy (Jones, 2009). According to Jones (2009) practitioners must be "aware of common cultural factors, such as direct and indirect communication styles within a cultural group, cultural differences between groups, knowledge of myths and stereotypes of a culture, and stressors associated with living in a multicultural context" (p. 194). In such an endeavor, practitioners must engage in collaboration with families to obtain accurate information about each adolescent's cultural history, including belief systems (Palacios & Trivedi, 2009). Once practitioners have endeavored this journey, they may work with other school staff in the process of working through, debunking stereotypes they hold, and initiating the process of developing cultural competency. Practitioners and school staff may also reach out to various Arab American organizations that provide cultural training to K-12 systems (Wingfield, 2006).

At the Tier I level, school-based mental health providers may work with school administrators in the implementation of anti-discrimination and anti-harassment policies when it comes to acts of bullying/harassment related to racial and religious biases (Tabbah et al., 2012). Ibish (2003) reported that schools that had such policies in place after 9/11 had significantly fewer incidents of discrimination. When it comes to the implementation of anti-bullying interventions, administrators must consider the cultural context, since many programs currently available have not been tested for efficacy within Arab American student populations (Haboush & Alyan, 2016). Future research may focus on investigating the effectiveness of established anti-bullying interventions with this population. Practitioners may help administrators identify key personnel within staff (i.e., educational psychologists, school psychologists, guidance counselors, school nurses, and teachers) in the reporting and intervention of such incidences (Tabbah, 2016). When a discriminatory event has been reported, practitioners may counsel the affected student and find out how the student has been impacted by the experience and connect them with the appropriate additional supports (Tabbah, Miranda, & Wheaton, 2016).

The literature calls for research examining Arab American students' self-perspectives of discrimination, bullying/harassment, and racial and religious biases in schools (Tabbah, Miranda, & Wheaton, 2016). Tabbah, Miranda, and Wheaton

(2016) suggested holding focus groups to interview students to gauge what they believe would be helpful to them in their schools and what could be possible solutions to combat discrimination and bullying. The authors speculate that this method may provide educators with valuable information, as well as a voice for Arab American adolescents. The information obtained from these groups can then be used in reforming school institutional policy for a more positive school climate.

As part of Tier I support services, Goforth et al. (2017) recommended universal mental health screening and the use of social-emotional curricula for Arab American students. Screening should involve both internalizing and externalizing behaviors in order for school-based mental health providers to determine if more intensive interventions are needed (e.g., Tier II). The authors emphasize the importance of screening given the mental health stigma prevalent in Arab American communities and that these youth may be at higher risk for internalizing problems (Aroian et al., 2009). Social-emotional curricula may be used to address internalizing and externalizing behavior issues for Arab American adolescents (Goforth et al., 2017).

Tier II involves students who are determined to be at-risk for mental health problems and require additional targeted and intensive interventions (Goforth et al., 2017). Goforth and colleagues recommended contacting the student's family when an Arab American student is determined to be at this level and then putting these additional supports into place. As discussed earlier in this chapter, keeping the family involved is critical in all areas of school-based services (Al Khateeb, Al Hadidi, & Al Khatib, 2015; Goforth et al., 2017). Other factors to keep in mind during this process are the collectivist and patriarchal nature of Arab American families, as well as family honor, where concerns that mental health issues may reflect poorly on the family (al-Krenawi & Graham, 2000). Goforth et al. (2017) recommended group counseling or interventions to address mental health issues with Arab American students at this tier level. It is important to remember issues with confidentiality that families may hold with concerns related to their children sharing information outside of the family. The authors noted that this may be especially true for students in ethnic enclaves where families know each other well and would be concerned that their children are sharing information with other children (Goforth et al., 2017). As discussed previously, then, it is critical for school-based mental health providers to emphasize the importance of confidentiality involved in group counseling (Goforth et al., 2017).

The research lacks studies regarding culturally relevant group treatment strategies for Arab American youth (Goforth et al., 2017). One peer support program was developed specifically for Arab American adolescents (Khouri, 2016). Khouri (2016) developed a program called the Circle Of Arab Students In Schools (see circleoasis.org), which is a group modality to help Arab students cope with stressors to help them be successful in life. The author reports that the program incorporates principles of rational emotive behavior therapy, positive psychology, and parts of the Resourceful Adolescent Program. Circle OASIS is implemented in peer groups consisting of four to six students and facilitated by a professional. There are two phases. The first phase is limited in time and implemented in ten sessions focusing on seven themes, including: (1) recognition and affirmation of personal strengths, (2) promoting self-management and self-regulation skills in the face of stress, (3) cognitive restructuring, (4) creating a personal problem-solving model, (5) building and accessing psychological support networks, (6) considering the other's perspective, and (7) keeping and making the peace. Then, the second phase is open ended and serves to help students practice the skills learned in the first phase along with issues they face daily. This program was created to help Arab American adolescents deal with the increasing animosity in American, as well as improve interpersonal skills and emotional intelligence (Khouri, 2016).

Goforth et al. (2017) also recommended assessing factors related to the process of acculturation, including acculturative stress associated with experiences of discrimination. Because adolescents under acculturative stress may be struggling with their identity as being Arab and/or American, it is critical for school-based mental health providers to screen for this through tier II level clinical interviews (Goforth et al., 2017). Goforth et al. (2017) suggested asking questions regarding the degree to which they identify with heritage and mainstream cultures, their comfort level with their native language, and affiliation with their heritage customs, values, and beliefs. School-based mental health professionals may then treat any symptoms associated with acculturative stress by teaching the student coping strategies to deal with identified symptoms (Goforth et al., 2017). Finally, school-based mental health providers may consider how to incorporate religious and cultural values into group counseling sessions (Goforth et al., 2017).

Tier III involves students who have been receiving Tier II services and have not improved in their mental health status and, therefore, require more intensive services or referral for special education services (Goforth et al., 2017). School-based mental health providers should conduct non-discriminatory assessments before providing services (Goforth et al., 2017) through a variety of procedures with an understanding of the student's ecological nature and contexts of learning (Ortiz, 2014). Providers should involve immediate and extended family members where relevant (Nassar-McMillan & Hakim-Larson, 2003), as well as consider cultural characteristics of the family and evaluate stigma they may hold regarding mental health (Goforth, 2011). In addition, when referral to special education services are warranted, school providers should clearly explain the process of special education to Arab American families (Al Khateeb et al., 2015), especially given the possible stigma families might hold regarding disabilities and special education in the Arab world discussed earlier in this chapter. Goforth et al. (2017) further recommended the consideration of personal or collective trauma in both assessment and treatment of Arab American students. For example, some families may have left their countries because of war, conflict, and/or oppression, which all contribute to trauma. The authors recommended delivery of multi-systemic and multi-modal interventions in these cases with account of family and community considerations in such treatment (Goforth et al., 2017).

Conclusion

Arab American cultures are severely misunderstood and portrayed negatively through the media in the United States. Consequently, Arab Americans face prejudice and discrimination from the mainstream public. Unfortunately, these views make their way into the schools and Arab American students have to cope with these perspectives along with discriminatory behaviors against them. An emerging body of research on Arab American youth provides evidence that discrimination experiences in the schools are related to developmental processes, including ethnic identity, self-concept, and mental health. The evidence demonstrates that various factors of the school environment need to be addressed.

Educators need to build cultural awareness and competence of Arab cultures and their students. The research showed that discrimination occurred from teachers as well as peers. Therefore, relationships with both groups need to be addressed. An increased cultural understanding by teachers and other school staff may facilitate more positive relationships with Arab students. Further, strategies may be implemented at all school levels to improve intergroup relationships between peers. Such activities may also improve educator relations with students.

Lack of representation and/or misrepresentation in curricula was a common theme across studies. Therefore, educational policy must focus on reforming curricula to include and accurately represent Arab cultures. The process for curriculum reform was presented relative to Arab cultures and students.

Finally, the research demonstrated negative relationships between school discrimination and developmental outcomes, including mental health. School-based mental health providers may follow an MTSS framework—with consideration of relevant cultural factors—to implement interventions appropriate for addressing identified issues. With culturally effective strategies for practice and policy in place, the K-12 system may potentially play a protective role in developmental processes of Arab American youth. These approaches, in combination, may help provide a safer and more inclusive school environment, which may then facilitate healthy development.

References

Abu El-Haj, T. R. (2006). Race, politics, and Arab American youth: Shifting frameworks for conceptualizing educational equity. *Educational Policy, 20*, 13–34. https://doi.org/10.1177/0895904805285287.

Abudabbeh, N. (2006). Arab families. In M. McGoldrick, J. Giordano, & J. K. Pearce (Eds.), *Ethnicity and family therapy* (2nd ed., pp. 333–346). New York: Guilford.

Aburumuh, H. A., Smith, H. L., & Ratcliffe, L. G. (2009). Educators' cultural awareness and perceptions of Arab-American students: Breaking the cycle of ignorance. *The Journal of Multiculturalism in Education, 4*. Retrieved from http://www.wtamu.edu/webres/File/Journals/MCJ/Volume4/aburumuh.pdf

Abu-saad, I. (1999). Self-esteem among Arab adolescents in Israel. *The Journal of Social Psychology, 139*(4), 479–486. https://doi.org/10.1080/00224549909598407.

Ahmed, S. R., Kia-Keating, M., & Tsai, K. H. (2011). A structural model of racial discrimination, acculturative stress, and cultural resources among Arab American adolescents. *American Journal of Community Psychology, 48*, 181–192. https://doi.org/10.1007/s10464-011-9424-3.

Ajrouch, K. J. (2000). Place, age, and culture: Community living and ethnic identity among Lebanese American adolescents. *Small Group Research, 31*(4), 447–469.

Al Khateeb, J. M., Al Hadidi, M. S., & Al Khatib, A. J. (2015). Addressing the unique needs of Arab American children with disabilities. *Journal of Child and Family Studies, 24*(8), 2432–2440. https://doi.org/10.1007/s10826-014-0046-x.

Al Lawati, S. (2011). Mentally disabled children in the Middle East and their integration into society. *Middle East Health*. Retrieved from http://www.middleeasthealthmag.com/cgi-bin/index.cgi?; http://www.middleeasthealthmag.com/jul2011/feature5.htm

Albdour, M., Lewin, L., Kavanaugh, K., Hong, J. S., & Wilson, F. (2017). Arab American adolescents' perceived stress and bullying experiences: A qualitative study. *Western Journal of Nursing Research, 39*(12), 1567–1588. https://doi.org/10.1177/0193945916678214.

Ali, S. R., Liu, W. M., & Humedian, M. (2004). Islam 101: Understanding the religion and therapy implications. *Professional Psychology: Research and Practice, 35*(6), 635–642. https://doi.org/10.1037/0735-7028.35.6.635.

Al-Khatab, A. (1999). In search of equity for Arab-American students in public schools of the United States. *Education, 120*, 254–266. Retrieved from http://proxy.lib.ohio-state.edu/login?url=http://search.ebscohost.com/login.aspx?direct=true&db=pbh&AN=2809113&site=ehost-live

al-Krenawi, A., & Graham, J. R. (2000). Culturally sensitive social work practice with Arab clients in mental health settings. *Health and Social Work, 25*(1), 9–22. https://doi.org/10.1093/hsw/25.1.9.

Al-Saffar, S., Borgå, P., Edman, G., & Hällström, T. (2003). The aetiology of posttraumatic stress disorder in four ethnic groups in outpatient psychiatry. *Social Psychiatry and Psychiatric Epidemiology, 38*(8), 456–462. https://doi.org/10.1007/s00127-003-0659-7.

Aroian, K., Hough, E. S., Templin, T. N., Kulwicki, A., Ramaswamy, V., & Katz, A. (2009). A model of mother–child adjustment in Arab Muslim immigrants to the US. *Social Science & Medicine, 69*(9), 1377–1386. https://doi.org/10.1016/j.socscimed.2009.08.027.

Arslan, H. (2009). Educational policy vs. culturally sensitive programs in Turkish educational system. *International Journal of Progressive Education, 5*(2), 44–57.

Artiles, A. J., & Ortiz, A. A. (2012). *English Language Learners with special education needs*. Retrieved from http://eric.ed.gov/?id=ED482995

Banks, J. A. (2003). *Teaching strategies for ethnic studies* (7th ed.). Boston, MA: Allyn and Bacon.

Barrett, M. (2007). *Children's knowledge, beliefs and feelings about nations and national groups*. Hove, England: Psychology Press/Taylor & Francis (UK).

Barrett, M. (2016). *Competencies for democratic culture: Living together as equals in culturally diverse democratic societies*. Retrieved from https://rm.coe.int/16806ccc07

Barrett, M. (2018). How schools can promote the intercultural competence of young people. *European Psychologist, 23*(1), 93–104. https://doi.org/10.1027/1016-9040/a000308.

Barrett, M., & Buchanan-Barrow, E. (2011). Children's understanding of society. In P. K. Smith & C. Hart (Eds.), *The Wiley-Blackwell handbook of childhood social development* (2nd ed., pp. 584–602). Chichester, UK: Blackwell-Wiley.

Barrett, M., Byram, M., Ipgrave, J., & Seurrat, A. (2013). *Images of others: An autobiography of intercultural encounters through visual media*. Retrieved from https://www.coe.int/en/web/autobiography-intercultural-encounters/images-of-others

Barrett, M., Byram, M., Lázár, I., Mompoint-Gaillard, P., & Philippou, S. (2013). *Developing intercultural competence through education*. Strasbourg, France: Council of Europe Publishing.

Benner, A. D., & Graham, S. (2013). The antecedents and consequences of racial/ethnic discrimination during adolescence: Does the source of discrimination matter? *Developmental Psychology, 49*(8), 1602–1613. https://doi.org/10.1037/a0030557.

Brittingham, A., & de la Cruz, G. P. (2005). *We the people of Arab ancestry in the United States: Census 2000 special reports*. United States Census Bureau. Retrieved from https://www.census.gov/prod/2005pubs/censr-21.pdf

Brown, C. S., & Chu, H. (2012). Discrimination, ethnic identity, and academic outcomes of Mexican immigrant children: The importance of school context. *Child Development, 83*(5), 1477–1485. https://doi.org/10.1111/j.1467-8624.2012.01786.x

Budman, C. L., Lipson, J. G., & Meleis, A. I. (1992). The cultural consultant in mental health care: The case of an Arab adolescent. *American Journal of Orthopsychiatry, 62*(3), 359–370. https://doi.org/10.1037/h0079347.

Byram, M., Barrett, M., Ipgrave, J., Jackson, R., & Méndez García, M. C. (2009). *Autobiography of intercultural encounters*. Retrieved from https://www.coe.int/en/web/autobiography-intercultural-encounters

Cameron, L., Rutland, A., Douch, R., & Brown, R. (2006). Changing children's intergroup attitudes toward refugees: Testing different models of extended contact. *Child Development, 77*(5), 1208–1219.

Carter, R. B., & El Hindi, A. E. (1999). Counseling Muslim children in school settings. *Professional School Counseling, 2*(3), 183–188.

Clotfelter, C. T. (2002). Interracial contact in high school extracurricular activities. *The Urban Review, 34*(1), 25–46. https://doi.org/10.1023/A:1014493127609.

Cohen, J., McCabe, L., Michelli, N. M., & Pickeral, T. (2009). School climate: Research, policy, practice, and teacher education. *Teachers College Record, 11*, 180–213. Retrieved from https://www.tcrecord.org/Content.asp?ContentId=15220

Crockett, D. P., & Brown, J. E. (2009). Multicultural practices and response to intervention. In J. M. Jones (Ed.), *The psychology of multiculturalism in the schools: A primer for practice, training, and research* (pp. 117–137). Bethesda, MD: National Association of School Psychologists.

de la Cruz, G. P., & Brittingham, A. (2003). *The Arab population: 2000. United States Census Bureau*. Retrieved from https://www.census.gov/prod/2003pubs/c2kbr-23.pdf

Deardorff, D. K. (2006). Identification and assessment of intercultural competence as a student outcome of internationalization. *Journal of Studies in International Education, 10*(3), 241–266. https://doi.org/10.1177/1028315306287002.

Devine, P. G., Forscher, P. S., Austin, A. J., & Cox, W. T. L. (2012). Long-term reduction in implicit bias: A prejudice habit-breaking intervention. *Journal of Experimental Social Psychology, 48*, 1267–1278. https://doi.org/10.1016/j.jesp.2012.06.003.

Dinero, S. C. (2002). Special education use among the Negev Bedouin Arabs of Israel: A case of minority under representation? *Race Ethnicity and Education, 5*(4), 377–396. https://doi.org/10.1080/1361332022000030897.

Duvdevany, I., & Abboud, S. (2003). Stress, social support and well-being of Arab mothers of children with intellectual disability who are served by welfare services in northern Israel. *Journal of Intellectual Disability Research, 47*(Pt 4–5), 264–272. https://doi.org/10.1046/j.1365-2788.2003.00488.x.

Dwairy, M., & Van Sickle, T. D. (1996). Western psychotherapy in traditional Arabic societies. *Clinical Psychology Review, 16*(3), 231–249. https://doi.org/10.1016/S0272-7358(96)00011-6.

Ebstyne King, P., & Furrow, J. L. (2004). Religion as a resource for positive youth development: Religion, social capital, and moral outcomes. *Developmental Psychology, 40*(5), 703–713. https://doi.org/10.1037/0012-1649.40.5.703.

El Naggar Gaad, E. (2001). Research section: Educating children with Down's syndrome in the United Arab Emirates. *British Journal of Special Education, 28*(4), 195–203. https://doi.org/10.1111/1467-8527.t01-1-00225.

Erickson, C. D., & Al-Timimi, N. R. (2001). Providing mental health services to Arab Americans: Recommendations and considerations. *Cultural Diversity and Ethnic Minority Psychology, 7*(4), 308–327.

Fisher, L., Evans, M., & Esch, E. (2004). Computer-mediated communication: Promoting learner autonomy and intercultural understanding at secondary level. *The Language Learning Journal, 30*(1), 50–58. https://doi.org/10.1080/09571730485200231.

Gaertner, S. L., & Dovidio, J. F. (2000). *Reducing intergroup bias: The common ingroup identity model*. New York: Psychology Press.

Gaines, A. D., & Farmer, P. E. (1986). Visible saints: Social cynosures and dysphoria in the mediterranean tradition. *Culture, Medicine and Psychiatry, 10*(4), 295–330. https://doi.org/10.1007/BF00049268.

Gay, G. (2000). *Culturally responsive teaching: Theory, research, & practice*. New York: Teachers College Press.

Goforth, A. N. (2011). Considerations for school psychologists working with Arab American children and families. *Communique, 32*(6), 1, 28, 30. Retrieved from http://www.nasponline.org/publications/periodicals/communique/issues/volume-39-issue-6/bmulticultural-affairsb-considerations-for-school-psychologists-working-with-arab-american-children-and-families

Goforth, A. N. (2016). A cultural humility model of school psychology training and practice. *Trainer's Forum, 34*, 3–24.

Goforth, A. N., Nichols, L. M., Stanick, C. F., Shindorf, Z. R., & Holter, O. (2017). School-based considerations for supporting Arab American youths' mental health. *Contemporary School Psychology, 21*(3), 191–200. https://doi.org/10.1007/s40688-016-0117-7.

Goforth, A. N., Oka, E. R., Leong, F. T. L., & Denis, D. J. (2014). Acculturation, acculturative stress, religiosity and psychological adjustment among Muslim Arab American adolescents. *Journal of Muslim Mental Health, 8*(2), 3–19. https://doi.org/10.3998/jmmh.10381607.0008.202.

Goforth, A. N., Pham, A. V., Chun, H., Castro-Olivo, S. M., & Yosai, E. R. (2016). Association of acculturative stress, Islamic practices, and internalizing symptoms among Arab American adolescents. *School Psychology Quarterly, 31*(2), 198–212. https://doi.org/10.1037/spq0000135.

Goforth, A. N., Pham, A. V., & Oka, E. R. (2015). Parent–child conflict, acculturation gap, acculturative stress, and behavior problems in Arab American adolescents. *Journal of Cross-Cultural Psychology, 46*(6), 821–836. https://doi.org/10.1177/0022022115585140.

Goode, T. (2002). *Self-assessment checklist for personnel providing services and supports to children and their families*. Retrieved from https://www.nasponline.org/resources-and-publications/resources/diversity/cultural-competence/self-assessment-checklist

Haboush, K. L. (2005). Lebanese and Syrian families. In M. McGoldrick, J. Giordano, & N. Garcia-Preto (Eds.), *Ethnicity and family therapy* (3rd ed., pp. 468–486). New York: Guilford Press.

Haboush, K. L. (2007). Working with Arab American families: Culturally competent practice for school psychologists. *Psychology in the Schools, 44*, 183–198. https://doi.org/10.1002/pits.20215.

Haboush, K. L., & Alyan, H. (2016). School psychology: Enhancing school climate and school connectedness. In M. M. Amer & G. H. Awad (Eds.), *Handbook of Arab American psychology* (pp. 318–330). New York: Routledge.

Haddad, S. (2002). Cultural diversity and sectarian attitudes in postwar Lebanon. *Journal of Ethnic and Migration Studies, 28*(2), 291–306. https://doi.org/10.1080/13691830220124341.

Hadidi, M. S. (1998). Educational services for visually impaired children in the Arab countries. *Journal of Visual Impairment & Blindness, 92*(7), 535–538. https://doi.org/10.1177/0145482x9809200714.

Hadidi, M. S., & Al Khateeb, J. M. (2015). Special education in Arab countries: Current challenges. *International Journal of Disability, Development and Education, 62*(5), 518–530. https://doi.org/10.1080/1034912X.2015.1049127.

Hakim-Larson, J., Kamoo, R., Nassar-McMillan, S. C., & Porcerelli, J. H. (2007). Counseling Arab and Chaldean American families. *Journal of Mental Health Counseling, 29*(4), 301–321. https://doi.org/10.17744/mehc.29.4.u5468716955w1023.

Hakim-Larson, J., & Menna, R. (2016). Acculturation and enculturation: Ethnic identity socialization process. In M. M. Amer & G. H. Awad (Eds.), *Handbook of Arab American psychology* (pp. 34–47). New York: Routledge.

Hamdi, E., Amin, Y., & Abou-Saleh, M. T. (1997). Problems in validating endogenous depression in the Arab culture by contemporary diagnostic criteria. *Journal of Affective Disorders, 44*(2–3), 131–143. https://doi.org/10.1016/s0165-0327(97)00037-2.

Hammer, M. R. (2004). *Assessment of the impact of the AFS study abroad experience*. New York: AFS Intercultural Programs.

Ibish, H. E. (2003). *Report on hate crimes and discrimination against Arab Americans: The post-September 11 Backlash September 11, 2001 - October 11, 2002*. Washington, DC: American Arab Anti-Discrimination Committee Research Institute.

Jones, J. M. (2009). Counseling with multicultural intentionality: The process of counseling and integrating client cultural variables. In J. M. Jones (Ed.), *The psychology of multiculturalism in the schools: A primer for practice, training, and research*. National Association of School Psychologists: Bethesda, MD.

Khouri, L. Z. (2016). On belonging: The American adolescent of Arab descent. *Journal of Clinical Psychology, 72*(8), 818–826. https://doi.org/10.1002/jclp.22363.

Kibbi, I. (1995). Lebanese and American educational differences: A comparison. *Education, 115*(3), 441–445.

Kulczycki, A., & Lobo, A. P. (2002). Patterns, determinants, and implications of intermarriage among Arab Americans. *Journal of Marriage and Family, 64*(1), 202–210. https://doi.org/10.1111/j.1741-3737.2002.00202.x.

Kumar, R., Karabenick, S. A., Warnke, J. H., Hany, S., & Seay, N. (2019). Culturally inclusive and responsive curricular learning environments (CIRCLEs): An exploratory sequential mixed-methods approach. *Contemporary Educational Psychology, 57*, 87–105. https://doi.org/10.1016/j.cedpsych.2018.10.005.

Kumar, R., Seay, N., & Karabenick, S. A. (2015). Immigrant Arab adolescents in ethnic enclaves: Physical and phenomenological contexts of identity negotiation. *Cultural Diversity and Ethnic Minority Psychology, 21*, 201–212. https://doi.org/10.1037/a0037748.

Kumar, R., Warnke, J. H., & Karabenick, S. A. (2014). Arab-American male identity negotiations: Caught in the crossroads of ethnicity, religion, nationality and current contexts. *Social Identities: Journal for the Study of Race, Nation and Culture, 20*(1), 22–41. https://doi.org/10.1080/13504630.2013.864464.

Ladson-Billings, G. (1992). Culturally relevant teaching: The key to making multicultural education work. In C. A. Grant (Ed.), *Research and multicultural education: From the margins to the mainstream* (pp. 106–121). Washington, DC: The Farmer Press.

Mackey, S. (1991). *Lebanon: Death of a nation*. New York: Doubleday.

Melhem, I., & Chemali, Z. (2014). Mental health of Arab Americans: Cultural considerations for excellence of care. In P. Ranna (Ed.), *The Massachusetts General Hospital textbook on diversity and cultural sensitivity in mental health* (pp. 3–30). Totowa, NJ: Humana Press.

Najjar, K., Naser, S. C., & Clonan-Roy, K. (2019). Experiences of Arab heritage youth in US schools and impact on identity development. *School Psychology International., 40*, 251. https://doi.org/10.1177/0143034319831057.

Nassar-McMillan, S. C., & Hakim-Larson, J. (2003). Counseling considerations among Arab Americans. *Journal of Counseling & Development, 81*(2), 150.

NEA. (2008). *Promoting educators' cultural competence to better serve culturally diverse students*. Washington, DC: NEA Human and Civil Rights Department.

Nobles, A. Y., & Sciarra, D. T. (2000). Cultural determinants in the treatment of Arab Americans: A primer for mainstream therapists. *American Journal of Orthopsychiatry, 70*(2), 182–191. https://doi.org/10.1037/h0087734.

Nydell, M. K. (2006). *Understanding Arabs: A guide for modern times* (4th ed.). Boston, MA: Intercultural Press.

Ortiz, S. (2014). Best practices in nondiscriminatory assessment. In P. L. Harrison & A. Thomas (Eds.), *Best practices in school psychology: Foundations* (pp. 661–678). Bethesda, MD: National Association of School Psychologists.

Palacios, E. D., & Trivedi, P. (2009). Increasing cultural literacy: Historical perspectives and cultural characteristics of minority groups. In J. M. Jones (Ed.), *The psychology of multiculturalism in the schools: A primer for practice, training, and research*. National Association of School Psychology: Bethesda, MD.

Pettigrew, T. F., & Tropp, L. R. (2006). A meta-analytic test of intergroup contact theory. *Journal of Personality and Social Psychology, 90*(5), 751–783. https://doi.org/10.1037/0022-3514.90.5.751.

Rhodes, R. L., Ochoa, S. H., & Ortiz, S. O. (2005). *Assessing culturally and linguistically diverse students: A practical guide*. New York: Guilford Press.

Sabry, N. S., & Bruna, K. R. (2007). Learning from the experience of Muslim students in American schools: Towards a proactive model of school-community cooperation. *Multicultural Perspectives, 9*(3), 44–50. https://doi.org/10.1080/15210960701443730.

Schwartz, W. (2002). *Arab American students in public schools*. Retrieved from https://www.adc.org/arab-american-students-in-public-schools/

Simmons, C., Simmons, C., & Habib Allah, M. (1994). English, Israeli-Arab and Saudi Arabian adolescent values. *Educational Studies, 20*(1), 69–86. https://doi.org/10.1080/0305569940200106.

Soueif, M. I., & Ahmed, R. A. (2001). Psychology in the Arab world: Past, present, and future. *International Journal of Group Tensions, 30*(3), 211–240. https://doi.org/10.1023/A:1011653930957.

Stathi, S., Cameron, L., Hartley, B., & Bradford, S. (2014). Imagined contact as a prejudice-reduction intervention in schools: The underlying role of similarity and attitudes. *Journal of Applied Social Psychology, 44*(8), 536–546. https://doi.org/10.1111/jasp.12245.

Stepick, A., & Stepick, C. D. (2002). Becoming American, constructing ethnicity: Immigrant youth and civic engagement. *Applied Developmental Science, 6*(4), 246–257. https://doi.org/10.1207/S1532480XADS0604_12.

Swindler Boutte, G., & Hill, E. L. (2006). African American communities: Implications for culturally relevant teaching. *The New Educator, 2*, 311–329.

Tabbah, R. (2016). The perils of Arab American adolescents post 9/11. *Journal for Multicultural Education, 10*(4), 449–464. https://doi.org/10.1108/JME-05-2015-0014.

Tabbah, R., Chung, J. J., & Miranda, A. H. (2016). Ethnic identity and discrimination: An exploration of the rejection-identification model in Arab American adolescents. *Identity, 16*(4), 319–334. https://doi.org/10.1080/15283488.2016.1231609.

Tabbah, R., Miranda, A. H., & Wheaton, J. E. (2012). Self-concept in Arab American adolescents: Implications of social support and experiences in the schools. *Psychology in the Schools, 49*, 817–827. https://doi.org/10.1002/pits.21640.

Tabbah, R., Miranda, A. H., & Wheaton, J. E. (2016). Intricacies of school relationships and the Well-being of Arab American youth: Implications for school psychologists. *Contemporary School Psychology, 20*(4), 315–326. https://doi.org/10.1007/s40688-016-0089-7.

Tabbah, R., Wheaton, J. E., & Miranda, A. H. (2015). Finding identity without discrimination: The plight of Arab American adolescents. *Identities: Global Studies in Culture and Power, 23*, 519–535. https://doi.org/10.1080/1070289X.2015.1064423.

Tatar, M., & Horenczyk, G. (2003). Dilemmas and strategies in the counselling of Jewish and Palestinian Arab children in Israeli schools. *British Journal of Guidance & Counselling, 31*(4), 375–391. https://doi.org/10.1080/03069880310001609268.

Turner, R. N., & Cameron, L. (2016). Confidence in contact: A new perspective on promoting cross-group friendship among children and adolescents. *Social Issues and Policy Review, 10*(1), 212–246. https://doi.org/10.1111/sipr.12023.

Turner, R. N., West, K., & Christie, Z. (2013). Out-group trust, intergroup anxiety, and out-group attitude as mediators of the effect of imagined intergroup contact on intergroup behavioral tendencies. *Journal of Applied Social Psychology, 43*(S2), E196–E205. https://doi.org/10.1111/jasp.12019.

UN. (2016). *Convention on the Rights of Persons with Disabilities-Articles*. Retrieved from https://www.un.org/development/desa/disabilities/convention-on-the-rights-of-persons-with-disabilities/convention-on-the-rights-of-persons-with-disabilities-2.html

UNESCO. (1994). *The Salamanca statement and framework for action on special needs education*. Retrieved from https://unesdoc.unesco.org/ark:/48223/pf0000098427

Weber, A. S. (2012). Inclusive education in the Gulf cooperation council. *Journal of Educational and Instructional Studies, 2*(2), 85–97.

Wingfield, M. (2006). Arab Americans: Into the multicultural mainstream. *Equity & Excellence in Education, 39*, 253–266. https://doi.org/10.1080/10665680600788453.

Wray-Lake, L., Syvertsen, A. K., & Flanagan, C. A. (2008). Contested citizenship and social exclusion: Adolescent Arab American immigrants' views of the social contract. *Applied Developmental Science, 12*, 84–92. https://doi.org/10.1080/10888690801997085.

Index

R. Tabbah, *Arab American Youth*, Advancing Responsible Adolescent Development, https://doi.org/10.1007/978-3-030-66804-4

The manufacturer's authorised representative in the EU is Springer Nature Customer Service Centre GmbH, Europaplatz 3, 69115 Heidelberg, Germany. If you have any concerns regarding our products, please contact ProductSafety@springernature.com

Printed and bound by CPI Group (UK) Ltd, Croydon, CR0 4YY
28/09/2026
02224088-0004